Using Nursing Case Management To Improve Health Outcomes

Michael Newell, RN, MSN, CCM
Consultant
Ernst & Young, LLP
Iselin, New Jersey

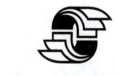

An Aspen Publication®
Aspen Publishers, Inc.
Gaithersburg, Maryland
1996

2.97

Library of Congress Cataloging-in-Publication Data

Newell, Michael.
Using nursing case management to improve
health outcomes / Michael Newell.
p.   cm.
Includes bibliographical references and index.
ISBN 0-8342-0623-4
1. Nursing care plans.   2. Nursing—Effect of managed care on.
3. Hospitals—Case management services.
I. Title.
RT49.N48   1996
362.1´73´068—dc 20
95-36702
CIP

Editorial Resources: Amy Myers-Payne

Library of Congress Catalog Card Number: 95-36702
ISBN: 0-8342-0623-4

Printed in the United States of America

1   2   3   4   5

To caregivers everywhere

Table of Contents

Foreword

The use of the case as an organizer of care delivery and research is both old and new. It has been most commonly used in practice venues that are person centered rather than disease centered. For example, management of the case is no stranger to public health nurses, psychiatric nurses in private practice, and occupational health nurses who managed the health of employees. Grand theories of human behavior have grown out of the study of collections of cases, Freud's neurotic patients, and Piaget's children. Case management has taken its rightful place as a care delivery method only recently as the health care system began to move from a parts-oriented focus to a whole-system focus, from fragmented to integrated managed care, and from acute care to primary care. Very simply, managing cases instead of visits or procedures makes better sense. Response to treatment, quality of life issues, and clinical outcomes can be documented and adjusted along the way while clients receive personal care.

Case management is a whole-system approach to care delivery rather than a parts-oriented approach. It focuses on the patient or family's responses to illness or trauma, and emphasizes empowerment rather than dependence on the system. Its appreciation of complexity promotes more targeted health outcomes, efficient care delivery, and cost-effectiveness. Case management in a managed-care environment can only be delivered by professionals who understand the nuances of health and illness, who can think on their feet, and who are challenged by working in environments of uncertainty.

Using Nursing Case Management To Improve Health Outcomes is a veritable "toolbox" for the would-be nurse case manager. This text explores the territory of case management as both a clinical and business tool, and specifies characteristics and requirements for effective case management. It incorporates the concept of case management within systems theory, and links it to continuous quality improvement methods and to the documentation of health outcomes. A nursing-oriented case management practice model is also provided. The model is user friendly. It details the components of case management that include not only the skill base but also those elements of the patient or family's support system that the case manager needs to engage. This book has a strong business component as well as an emphasis on ethical approaches to care.

The author, Michael Newell, is an expert in and practitioner of case management and it shows. The cases are real, the skill base for case management is well specified, and the issues involved in conducting case management in a managed-care environment are clearly delineated. Furthermore, the organization of this book is both simple and elegant. It guides the reader into grappling with the system, the patient, and finally the future where case management will be a dominant method of care delivery.

—Gloria F. Donnelly, PhD, RN, FAAN
Dean and Professor
School of Nursing
La Salle University
Philadelphia, Pennsylvania

Preface

Nursing case management has evolved from an insurance and business perspective. It has therefore been difficult for many clinicians to understand how it can be used in all the various settings seen now. The effective use of case management has suffered from misconceptions about what it is, when it should be used, and how it fits with nursing (and other) clinical practice.

The purpose of this book is

1. to provide a broad overview of the various settings and forms of case management
2. to present a theoretical model of case management congruent with nursing and general systems theory
3. to indicate the skill sets and training needs required for nurses to be successful case managers
4. to show how case management is congruent with quality improvement (QI) theory
5. to review health outcomes measures so as to assist case managers in determining who should be case managed and to determine the appropriateness, effectiveness, and efficiency of proposed medical and rehabilitative interventions
6. to provide an ethical framework for case managers that goes beyond the justice/beneficence model that has been largely inadequate

7. to provide some tools for patient-focused goal setting that can enable the patient and family to be their own case managers
8. to indicate the complexities and variety of case management practice through the case examples provided
9. to identify what types of activities case managers perform, so as to assist in professional development and preparation for certification (CCM, or certified case manager)
10. to provide a vision of the future possibilities of case management as changes in the reimbursement, technology, and societal expectations influence the practice of health care

Case management practice is evolving faster and in more directions than anyone would have dreamed a short time ago. As insurance companies and the other payers of health services are seeing, health services are much more efficient and effective if they are rendered in a coherent fashion. Nursing case management brings this coherence to the patient and is so far a largely untapped resource to promote superior health outcomes to patients in virtually any setting.

—*Michael Newell, RN, MSN, CCM*

Acknowledgments

I would like to thank my wife, Nadia, for her patience. And thank you to my family, and the extended family of nurses who find ways to care for others that are unique and wondrous. I would especially like to thank the following nurses: Suzanne Adams, Jane Dias, Christine Rosenheim, Bob Hess, and Wendie Hunt, who first hired me to be a case manager.

—*M.N.*

Part I

Engaging the System

1

Defining Case Management: A Theoretical Framework

Case management is a multidisciplinary process that seeks to support and guide patients throughout their health encounter. The definition of *case management* worked out by the Individual Case Management Association (ICMA) and the Case Management Society of America (CMSA) is as follows: "Case management is a collaborative process which assesses, plans, implements, coordinates, monitors and evaluates options and services to meet an individual's health needs through communication and available resources to promote quality, cost-effective outcomes."[1] Case management has evolved in accordance with the requirements of the payer of health benefits, which is to say it has been structured to meet the cost containment and utilization management needs of the insurance plan involved. Cost containment strategies have been related to

1. structuring benefits; excluding high-risk individuals, discovering those with pre-existing conditions
2. coordinating the care of catastrophic claims or chronic patients
3. performing retrospective utilization review on unusual or high-dollar cases.

Defining *case management* is a difficult task because there are so many settings in which some variation of case management is practiced. Definitions of *case management* are scattered across the social work, insurance, mental health, nursing, and medical literature. Primary care physicians and specialty practice physicians feel that they do case management, and there is a long tradition of it among social workers, primarily for clients with nonmedical problems. Nurses make up 90 percent of case managers in private rehabilitation, indemnity insurance, preferred provider organizations (PPOs), the medical portion of workers' compensation claims, and most health maintenance organizations (HMOs). Social workers are used in long-term care, general human services care, psychiatric settings, and some (mostly older, group-model) HMOs, although many nurses are now active in such settings as well. M.S.W.s generally manage the vocational assessment and placement component of workers' compensation claims.

Case managers who operate outside a provider institution or setting are called *external* case managers, or *large* case managers, because they handle high-dollar or complex cases that need oversight and/or coordination. Many of these case managers are agents of insurance companies and practice from the payer's point of view. Others are agents for case management companies or lawyers or are company occupational health nurses.

Case managers who operate within provider institutions, such as hospitals, long-term care facilities, HMOs, and home care agencies, are referred to as *internal* case managers because they are part of the treatment team. Their role has to do with tracking utilization of resources, coordinating care, and communicating with payers, families, and service providers beyond the scope of their employer. Chapter 2 provides a more in-depth discussion of the varied settings of case management.

For the purposes of simplicity, this book defines case managers as nurses. Although social workers do medical case management in some settings and with some high-risk populations, their efficacy has been questioned due to their lack of medical training.[2] Our view is that nurses are the most appropriately trained professional personnel to provide case management.

Because nursing has traditionally valued multidisciplinary efforts that are client focused, this book also defines case management in terms of nursing theory. Such theory takes a systems perspective of person, environment, health, and nursing, and attempts to specify the relationships between them so that some day it may be put to the test of research: systemization, control, empiricism, and critical review.[3]

MODELS OF HEALTH AND ILLNESS

Much of the discussion on health care reform has focused on the insurance, financing, and costs of health care.[4] Fundamental reform, however, must involve a shift from a strictly biomedical perspective on health and illness to a broader systems approach. A systems framework for viewing the health of human populations would offer an orientation to complexity—a way to see the whole and the parts within it. It would offer some analytic techniques for sorting out relationships and solving problems and some organizing constructs that would model real-life situations.[5]

The inadequacy of the biomedical model and the need for a general systems theory in health care have been recognized since the 1970s.[6] In 1977, Engel published a critique of the biomedical model in *Science*.[7] This model, as he described it, was reductionist in that it sought single causes of disease and separated the mental and the somatic. Although this method had been useful at the beginning of the scientific revolution, it had now become dogma defended by vested interests. Any data that did not fit the model were excluded.

Engel proposed a *biopsychosocial* model of disease. This model would take into account the patient, the social context in which he or she lived, and the societal system designed to deal with the disruptive effects of illness. Engel split the definition of *illness* from that of *disease*. *Disease* is a biomedical term; *illness* encompasses the patient's self-reported symptoms as well as functional, psychological, and social manifestations.

Engel's biopsychosocial model would enable healers to deal with the many instances in which patients do not know what is wrong or feel incapable of helping themselves. Engel stated that "the critical factor underlying man's need to develop folk models of disease, and to develop social adaptations to deal with the individual and group disruptions brought about by the disease, has always been the victim's ignorance of what is responsible for his dysphoric or disturbing symptoms."[8]

Figure 1–1 shows Engel's model of a hierarchy of systems, each of which is a component of a higher system.[9] The place of the individual human being in this model is at the top of the organismic hierarchy and at the bottom of the social hierarchy.

More recently, and along similar lines, Pawlson stated that the prevailing model for health care delivery is the acute-simple-disease model (see Figure 1–2). This model assumes a single cause for a biologic disease that prompts a technical intervention by hospital-centered subspecialists who focus on a physiologic endpoint called a "cure."[10] The acute-simple-disease model assumes that patients are passive recipients of care and that interventions outside the mechanistic worldview of allopathic medicine have little to offer.

Given, however, that 80 percent of health care resources in the United States are devoted to chronic disease,[11] this form of care seems poorly suited to current needs. The medical treatment given in the United States

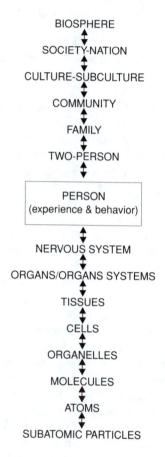

Figure 1–1 Hierarchy of Natural Systems

may be the most technically complex and proficient, but is the care appropriate? The acute-simple-disease model has created our present quandary with respect to the financing and delivery of care. In short, this model has been dysfunctional for a long time.

In this book we use the term *medical care* to describe an approach to dealing with bodily injury and somatic complaints that is based on the acute-simple-disease model. Medical care is a profession-dominated enterprise that has defined the needs for the customer (patients, payers,

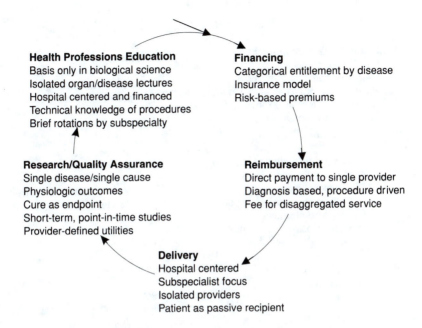

Health Professions Education
Basis only in biological science
Isolated organ/disease lectures
Hospital centered and financed
Technical knowledge of procedures
Brief rotations by subspecialty

Financing
Categorical entitlement by disease
Insurance model
Risk-based premiums

Research/Quality Assurance
Single disease/single cause
Physiologic outcomes
Cure as endpoint
Short-term, point-in-time studies
Provider-defined utilities

Reimbursement
Direct payment to single provider
Diagnosis based, procedure driven
Fee for disaggregated service

Delivery
Hospital centered
Subspecialist focus
Isolated providers
Patient as passive recipient

Figure 1–2 Acute-Simple-Disease Model. *Source*: Reprinted from Pawlson, L.G., Chronic Illness: Implications of a New Paradigm for Health Care, *Joint Commission Journal on Quality Improvement*, Vol. 20, No. 1, pp. 33–42, with permission of Mosby-Year Book, © 1994.

society) and holds itself to be the evaluator of quality. In contrast, we use the term *health care* to describe care that is based on the chronic-complex-illness model. The chronic-complex-illness model (see Figure 1–3) is a more appropriate model for health care delivery.[12] Multiple contributing biopsychosocial factors cause an illness that has no clear-cut etiology or cure and that has fluctuating and sometimes unpredictable levels of symptom severity (see Figure 1–4). Caretaker and patient must engage in a continuous process to limit functional losses and relieve the suffering. The patient and family assume an active role. The payers and providers assume a risk-sharing relationship.

Prevention, coordination, and nonmedical interventions have added value. A quality outcome for the patient is defined in terms of patient- and society-defined utilities: functional health, feeling of well-being, and satisfaction with how one is treated (caring). The most appropriate caregivers are those trained in the social, behavioral, and biological sciences. The most appropriately educated and socialized caregivers in the chronic-complex-illness model are professional nurses.

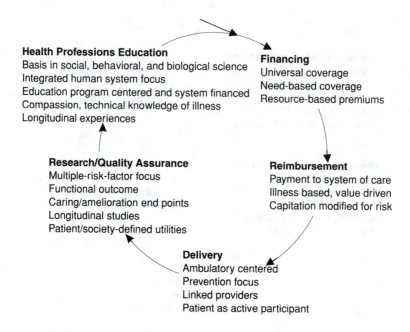

Health Professions Education
Basis in social, behavioral, and biological science
Integrated human system focus
Education program centered and system financed
Compassion, technical knowledge of illness
Longitudinal experiences

Financing
Universal coverage
Need-based coverage
Resource-based premiums

Research/Quality Assurance
Multiple-risk-factor focus
Functional outcome
Caring/amelioration end points
Longitudinal studies
Patient/society-defined utilities

Reimbursement
Payment to system of care
Illness based, value driven
Capitation modified for risk

Delivery
Ambulatory centered
Prevention focus
Linked providers
Patient as active participant

Figure 1–3 Chronic-Complex-Illness Model. *Source*: Reprinted from Pawlson, L.G., Chronic Illness: Implications of a New Paradigm for Health Care, *Joint Commission Journal on Quality Improvement*, Vol. 20, No. 1, pp. 33–42, with permission of Mosby-Year Book, © 1994.

NURSING THEORY

Foundations of Nursing Theory: Florence Nightingale

The declared purpose of Florence Nightingale's 1859 treatise *Notes on Nursing: What It Is, What It Is Not*[13] is "to give hints for thought to women who have personal charge of the health of others."[14] The central theoretical proposition is that the laws of health and nursing apply among the well as among the sick, and that nursing "ought to signify the proper use of fresh air, light, warmth, cleanliness, quiet and the proper selection and administration of diet—all at the least expense to the vital power of the patient."[15] Thus nursing's primary concern is the interaction between the patient and his or her environment.

Nightingale's systematic description of the phenomena of disease and nursing still resonates with a clarity of purpose and a focus on process over structure. Her intuitive grounded-theory approach[16] emphasizes explanation and understanding of phenomena, using one important assumption: that disease is part of God's "reparative" process, the symptoms of which

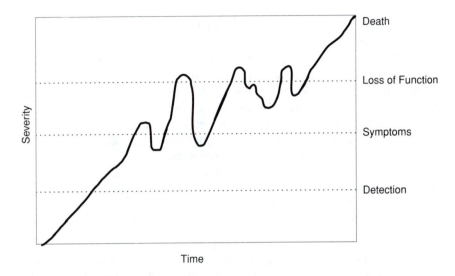

Figure 1–4 The Complex Path of Chronic Illness. *Source:* Reprinted from Pawlson, L.G., Chronic Illness: Implications of a New Paradigm for Health Care, *Joint Commission Journal of Quality Improvement*, Vol. 20, No. 1, pp. 33–42, with permission of Mosby-Year Book, © 1994.

may abate (or can at least be better defined) if the above mentioned essentials are provided. Nightingale explored in her work the basic human disposition to find meaning in events (especially sickness/injury/death events) that affect one's life. She accepted what we would now call a symbolic interactionalist worldview in that she was interested in how people ascribe meaning to illness and act out learned roles when faced with illness.

Nightingale coded her data into categories and basic social processes much as grounded theorists do, without the benefit of other scientific or descriptive literature to assist her. She was a participant observer of thousands of sick and wounded people in battlefield hospitals, at home, and in the hospitals of her day. The content of her book is theory generating because she used ideas from her lived experience to speak to the health policy issues of the day (e.g., criticizing the equation of hospital building with health status).[17]

Human Beings as Behavioral Systems: Dorothy Johnson

Dorothy Johnson used Nightingale's statement that nursing's primary concern is the interaction between the patient and his or her environment as a starting point for her theoretical construct of human beings as behavioral systems.[18] Human behavioral systems, taking our cue from Engle, interact with their external environment, but also interact with their internal systems, each of which has its own operational environment. These environments require nurturing in order to achieve optimal functioning. Human beings need to be listening and responding to the messages from within their bodies (their internal environments) if they are to heal the wounds of illness and injury. Case managers need to be aware of the effects of external and internal environments on the functioning of human systems. For Johnson, each human being is a behavioral system made up of all patterned, repetitive, and purposeful ways of behavior.[19] Seven subsystems carry out specialized tasks to maintain the whole behavioral system and manage the environment:

1. *attachment or affiliative*—attainment of security needs for survival, social inclusion, intimacy, and formation and maintenance of social bonds
2. *dependency*—succoring behavior that calls for nurturance, approval, attention, recognition, and physical assistance
3. *ingestive*—appetite satisfaction in reference to eating, respiration, and to social and psychological hungers such as touching and conversing functions
4. *eliminative*—control of when, how, and under what conditions body waste is eliminated
5. *sexual*—procreation and gratification with regard to behaviors; biologic sex, including courting and mating
6. *aggressive*—protection and preservation of self and society
7. *achievement*—control of some aspect of self or environment in reference to intellectual, physical, creative, mechanical, social, and caretaking skills

Johnson defined nursing in systems theory terms as directed toward controlling the system's functioning at certain critical points where it is out of balance. The goal is to restore and maintain balance and stability at the highest possible level for the individual.[20] Nursing intervention involves imposing temporary external regulatory or control mechanisms on behavior, changing the structural elements of the subsystem, and fulfilling the subsystem's functional requirements.

Although the subsystems that Johnson proposed are behaviorally oriented, they are not amenable to use in daily practice. Other constructs that she developed, however, are broadly applicable to the work of all caregivers.

Johnson stated that human systems consist of four structural elements:

1. *drive*—toward goals; motivation is inferred by observation of behavior
2. *set*—a predisposition to act in certain ways to fulfill functional subsystems
3. *choice*—the total repertoire of behavioral patterns that hopefully fulfill the subsystems' functions
4. *action*—directly observable behavior

In addition, human systems have three *functional requirements:*

1. no noxious influences that prevent coping
2. nurturance through input of appropriate supplies from the environment
3. stimulation to enhance growth

Johnson saw nursing as assisting people in fulfilling their system's functional requirements when they are unable to do so, by giving protection, nurturance, and stimulation via external regulatory measures.

Johnson believed that three types of knowledge are required for the practice of nursing:

1. *knowledge of order*—assumption that there is order in nature and that this order is discoverable; scientific knowledge and knowledge of normal human functioning and behavior
2. *knowledge of disorder*—understanding of events that pose a threat to the well-being of a person or society
3. *knowledge of control*—knowledge enabling one to carry out a prescribed course of action to reach a desired outcome

Johnson's constructs are useful for case managers in that they focus on ways to assist clients with health-related issues. By understanding human beings as behavioral systems that have structural elements and functional requirements, case managers can better understand and assist clients and patients to make choices and take actions that will fulfill their needs. External regulatory measures that interact with institutional and human systems are required for success in meeting treatment goals. The case manager's understanding of order, disorder, and control issues in health care, social service, legal, insurance, and human behavioral systems can assist in constructing action (treatment or care) plans that are oriented to the patient's health, functional, and spiritual needs.

A PRACTICE MODEL OF CASE MANAGEMENT

This book is based on a "practice model" of case management to guide the practitioner in selecting the most effective means of obtaining a quality health outcome. This model, shown in Figures 1–5 and 1–6, encompasses activities that revolve around the patient and family and is configured as a wheel to suggest movement forward regarding patient goals.

In Figure 1–5, the case management wheel places the patient and family (or close community of support) at the center of a system of human interaction. The case manager brings to the process the skill sets that are depicted as the spokes of the wheel. Training in *systems theory* and functioning, in *negotiation* and facilitation skills, and *communication* skills, including people skills, training, and facility with information systems, is very important.

Care coordination skills come with practice and support of all parties. An *ethic of caring* that includes all parties to a negotiated process or plan of care (not just treatment) needs to be taught and valued. In an age of limited resources, all generations and communities of solution need to reassess their values when engaged in the health care system. Case managers need to be trained and supported to assist with these issues.

Reporting and evaluation (another way of saying "collection of outcomes data") have always been a major part of the case manager's job. This task will become much more important, triggering additional training needs for case managers.

Coaching skill goes along with negotiation, communication, and coordination as a requirement of a successful case manager. It may be the highest "value-added" service that a case manager can provide.

Clinical expertise will be very valuable for case managers, especially internal case managers who follow patients through critical pathways. Case managers who can handle patients with chronic conditions and multiple comorbid factors will be highly valued.

The wheel in Figure 1–6 shows how various classifications of involved entities should be relating to the patient and family. *Primary care physicians* have an incentive to cooperate with the case manager concerning the small subset of patients who have triggered case management involvement. Such involvement lowers physicians' resource use and generally makes their life easier.

Public health initiatives, including state and federal surveillance, research and funding activity, and laws and regulations, are coordinated to mesh with the private sector. This power counterbalances that of the dominant contractors and deliverers of care, the *managed-care organizations*.

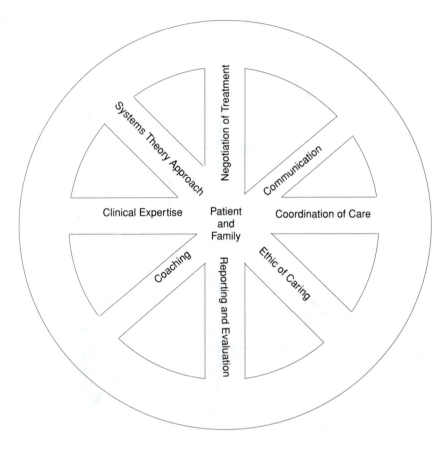

Figure 1–5 A Case Management Practice Model

A special place is given to the *spiritual* support system, which is in-volved in care delivery as directed by the patient, the family, and the extended support group or interest group, the *community of solution*. The *legal* support system, including standards of care and other methods of ensuring quality, should assist with the process of contracting fairly for services. It should be able to assist with end-of-life arrangements and other adjudication as the health care system moves through "reform."

The *employer* of the patient also has rights and responsibilities in the system. The well-being of the employee should be in his or her best interest. Self-insurance incentives and coherent occupational safety and workers' compensation systems are essential to a well-functioning health care system.

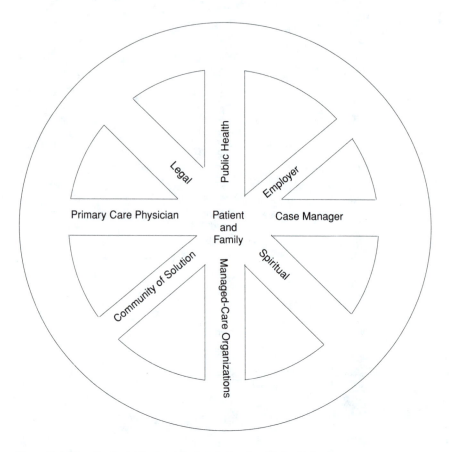

Figure 1–6 How the Social Support System Interacts with the Patient

The model is designed to fit the multiple areas in which nurses and others practice case management. It is easy to understand, and it allows practitioners to control (or at least negotiate control over) their everyday situations. Our view is that *case management systems must act like well-functioning human systems* if we are to take advantage of the opportunity to provide quality, cost-effective health care. Case management systems must act like human beings that are well functioning: They are focused on the task at hand, interact without duplicity, they learn and respond to new situations and information, they are honest and forthright in communicating with all parties. Well-functioning case managers and case management systems may not always do everything right, but they should strive to do the right thing, thus affecting others in the system to also act with integrity.

Case management, being a component of managed care, fits well with the "shared-risk" model of true managed care.[21] Shared risk involves providers and payers in reimbursement arrangements that should lead to greater efficiency in terms of resource use (e.g., capitated payment). Under shared risk, all participants (payer, provider, and patient) are at risk if the process of health delivery is not carried out with technical efficiency and fairness. This rationale presupposes that the provider will practice ethically and not withhold or deny care when it is required. It assumes that the patient has no hidden agendas or secondary gains from the disease, and it also assumes that the managed care organization's policies are consistent, fair, and honest in conception and practice.

Patients are sharing risk in that they take the chance that the provider of care is looking after their best interests. Patients who are involved in case management should be engaged in a system that requires them to play (to the best of their ability) an active part in formulating their plan of care. This structural control technique enables the plan of care to be appropriate to the goals of the patient. All parties have an incentive to keep the plan of care on track.

The essence of continuous quality improvement (CQI)/total quality management (TQM) theory (we will use *QI* for short to mean both) is to get feedback from both internal and external customers by responding sensitively to their needs. *Case management done properly is the essence of QI.* All those involved in a patient's care are customers, and it makes sense for care managers to have the requisite psychosocial skills, training, and tradition, as nurses do. Nursing case management can be very rewarding when it is working well, with marvelous results for patient health outcomes.[22] It can be the most fully considered and effective way to institutionalize caring in this society.

Case management, then, is a system of care that helps the sick and the well to learn and behave in a way that enables them to cope with the challenges of their illness event. This book presents examples and scenarios of the when, what, and how of case management.

NOTES

1. Case Management Society of America, CMSA Proposes Standards of Practice, *The Case Manager* 5, no. 1 (1994): 60.

2. E. Sampson, The Emergence of Case Management Models, in *Outpatient Case Management: Strategies for a New Reality*, ed. M.R. Donovan and T.A. Matson (Chicago: American Hospital Publishing, 1994), 85.

3. J. Fawcett, The Relationship between Theory and Research: The Double Helix, in *Perspective on Nursing Theory*, ed. L. Nicoli (Boston: Little, Brown & Co., 1986).

4. T.A. Brennan, An Ethical Perspective on Health Insurance Reform, *American Journal of Law and Medicine* 19, nos. 1 and 2 (1993):37–74.

5. A. Sheldon et al., Current Issues in Systems and Medical Care, in *Systems and Medical Care*, ed. A. Sheldon et al. (Cambridge, Mass.: MIT Press, 1970), 329–331.

6. F. Baker, General Systems Theory, Research and Medical Care, in *Systems and Medical Care*, ed. A. Sheldon et al. (Cambridge, Mass.: MIT Press, 1970), 1–26.

7. G.L. Engel, The Need for a New Medical Model: A Challenge for Biomedicine, *Science* 196 (1977):129–136.

8. Engel, Need for a New Medical Model, 133.

9. G.L. Engel, The Clinical Application of the Biopsychosocial Model, *American Journal of Psychiatry* 137 (1980):535–544.

10. L.G. Pawlson, Chronic Illness: Implications of a New Paradigm for Health Care, *Joint Commission Journal on Quality Improvement* 20, no. 1 (1994):33–42.

11. L.E. Cluff, Chronic Disease, Function and the Quality of Care, *Journal of Chronic Diseases* 34 (1981):299–304.

12. Pawlson, Chronic Illness, 36.

13. F. Nightingale, *Notes on Nursing: What It Is, What It Is Not* (London: Harrison, 1859), preface.

14. Nightingale, *Notes on Nursing*, preface.

15. Nightingale, *Notes on Nursing*, 6.

16. Western Nursing Research Society, *Guidelines for Reviewing Qualitative Research* (1987).

17. I.B. Cohen, Florence Nightingale, *The Smithsonian*, March 1984, 128–137.

18. D. Wallace (producer) and T. Coberg (director), *Portraits of Excellence: Dorothy Johnson*, Oakland, Calif., Studio Three, 1988.

19. D.E. Johnson, The Behavioral System Model for Nursing, in *Conceptual Models for Nursing*, 2nd ed., ed. J.P. Riehl and C. Roy, Sr. (New York: Appleton & Lange, 1980), 206–216.

20. Wallace and Coberg, *Portraits of Excellence*.

21. A.L. Hillman et al., Contractual Arrangements between HMOs and Primary Care Physicians: Three-Tiered HMOs and Risk Pools, *Medical Care* 30, no. 2 (1992):136–148.

22. Institute of Medicine, *Controlling Costs and Changing Patient Care: The Role of Utilization Management*, ed. B. Gray and M. Field (Washington, D.C.: National Academy Press, 1989), 130–138.

2

Areas of Case Management

EXTERNAL CASE MANAGEMENT

External case management, which includes brokered and episodic case management,[1] also called *outpatient case management*,[2] encompasses management activity that is external to provider organizations. The case manager coordinates, coaxes, and counsels patient, family, provider, and payer toward identified goals. This activity is also called *large case management* by indemnity, self-funded, and "stop-loss" insurers and third-party administrators.

The case manager gets involved on a case-by-case basis with patients who have a catastrophic injury or illness or who have reached a dollar threshold that triggers the need for a knowledgeable clinician to review the case and offer alternatives to the treatment plan. The primary motivation of the insurance company is to save money, but sometimes insurance companies use case managers to provide a higher level of service to important client organizations or claimants.

The ability of the case manager to recommend and carry out strategies of cost containment is contingent on

- the type of insurance coverage
- exclusions in the policy

- the ability of the case manager to handle patients, families, and other interested parties (e.g., lawyers, state social workers) to coordinate activities and treatment plans
- knowledge the case manager may have concerning alternative funding sources for medical benefits, such as Medicaid waiver programs, coverage for brain-injured children under Individuals with Disabilities Education Act (IDEA) laws, or rare disease research and treatment trials
- the ability of the case manager to discover other coverages that may be relevant and may stretch benefit dollars, using secondary or subrogated carriers (see "Coordination of Benefits" section in Chapter 4)
- the willingness of the insurance company to consider alternative treatment plans that may not be specifically covered, called out-of-contract arrangements

External case managers need to have a working knowledge of provisions of various types of insurance coverage, as well as clinical expertise regarding the type of case in which they are involved. Ideally, they should also have access to information on alternative coverages to coordinate benefits.

Although many insurance companies have their own rehabilitation or case management nurses on staff, they sometimes find it beneficial to contract for case management with individual case management companies instead of using their own employees. Individual case management companies, which have flourished since the late 1970s, are often used to coordinate catastrophic injury auto cases, to handle burgeoning workers' compensation claims, and to perform various retrospective utilization review functions. Reasons for delegating this work to an outside vendor include efficiency in handling peaks in the workload, absence of on-site capability where the claimant lives, special expertise of the case management vendor, and an "arm's-length" relationship between the external case manager and the insurance company. Although this tactic may be somewhat inefficient as a rule, it gives claimants and lawyers some incentive to cooperate if the case manager can present him- or herself in a mediator role.

Individual case managers are also hired by personal injury and workers' compensation lawyers and by insurance companies that want them to do retrospective bill audits or other utilization review tasks, including setting up peer reviews and independent medical exams (IMEs). The following are various areas of external case management.

Catastrophic Auto Claims

Catastrophically injured victims of motor vehicle accidents tend to have the benefit of case management when the coverage is substantial and the insurance carrier wishes to produce a sentinel effect on the various providers. Case managers encourage early discharge from acute care to rehabilitation and to home, which not only saves benefit dollars but has been shown to improve functional outcomes of selected patients (e.g., those with head injuries).[3] They also get involved in decisions regarding discharge planning to home, adaptive equipment, and home modification.

Chronically injured auto claimants also trigger case management involvement, especially if questionable provider bills and/or obstructive personal injury lawyers seem to be involved. Case managers set up IMEs, sometimes attending the examinations in order to ensure that pertinent questions are answered concerning pre-existing conditions, levels of pain and function, and the appropriateness of the treatment plan. The case manager generally performs the following tasks:

1. *Chart review/assessment*: The case manager reviews the claims history and file in order to determine whether the care and documentation are appropriate and whether the claim is worth case managing.
2. *Peer review*, done to determine the appropriateness of the care rendered and the charges: The case manager sends provider documentation and bills to a physician who is from the same subspecialty and asks him or her to determine whether the treatment plan and charges are appropriate.
3. *IME*: The case manager sends the treatment plan progress notes and billing history to a doctor, who examines the patient to give a determination (more authoritative than a peer review) as to whether the care rendered was appropriate. The IME provider may be asked to suggest an alternative treatment plan or, on rare occasions, to take over the care of a patient. Generally, IME physicians are not expected to gain from the review. The best IME physicians are board certified in their subspecialty. Reviewers are ranged on a hierarchy of authority: for example, a neurosurgeon may be asked to determine whether a laminectomy done by an orthopedist is appropriate, or a physiatrist may be asked to render an opinion on rehab care given by a general practitioner.

Workers' Compensation

Workers' compensation statutes differ from state to state, but they generally provide the exclusive remedy for an employee injured on the job. Workers' compensation is a social contract by state governments that mandates "first-dollar" or total coverage of medical bills and a percentage of lost wages for on-the-job injuries or illness. Injured employees are precluded from recovering from their employer or coemployees for negligence or other claims apart from the workers' compensation claim.[4]

Case management ideally begins at the time of the first report of injury. Although the majority of injuries do not require case management, some kind of timely risk management review is helpful in (1) establishing the genuineness, cause, and extent of the injury; and (2) demonstrating to the employee that there is some agent from the employer who cares about the individual as a person and who may be monitoring the actions of the parties involved.

Such a course of action requires an integrated disability management strategy on the part of the employer and insurance entity. It is logistically easier for self-insured employers who have contracted with a panel of health providers to carry out such a holistic strategy. Usually such forward-thinking integrated response structures have been established by larger employers who have certain classifications of employees at risk for certain types of injuries. The high-technology employers have been proactive in this regard, with good results (see the example of Honeywell in the section "Occupational Health Nursing" later in this chapter), but they are struggling with newer types of injury patterns, such as repetitive motion (e.g., carpal tunnel syndrome) and psychiatric stress disorders.

Many states have vocational rehabilitation training and placement structured into their workers' compensation laws, although many provisions for vocational rehab have been relaxed by law revisions in more recent years. This is because the vocational component tends to drive up the costs of workers' compensation insurance and has been shown to be of little value, especially when the economy is in a depressed cycle.

Case management goals are to return the claimant to his or her previous state of health or to a condition of maximum medical improvement (MMI). The case manager seeks to ensure that the treatment plan is appropriate and progressive, that the claimant is compliant with the treatment regimen, and that the claimant is not engaged in any activities that would jeopardize his or her recovery.

The general rule of thumb is that if an injured worker is not back to work within six months of injury, there is only a 50 percent chance that he or she will return. A year of work loss drops the return rate to 25 percent, with the return-to-work rate dropping to near zero after two years off the job.[5] This is because so many workers learn to accommodate themselves to a lower wage rate and an unemployed lifestyle during this period. Some claimants find "under-the-table" wages in another industry and have no incentive to return to their former job or a lower paying position.

Knowledge Requirements for Workers' Compensation by Case Managers

Case managers who work with workers' compensation claimants need to be familiar with the law in their state and need to assess the motivation of the claimant to return to work. How does the injury episode affect the claimant's self-esteem? Does he or she verbalize motivation to return to his or her employer, or is he or she angry or evasive? Does the claimant have a family to support? Does he or she engage in high-risk behaviors or substance abuse? Does the claimant have transferable skills that will enable him or her to adapt to modified job opportunities? The role of the employer in smoothing the way back to work and thus limiting the payout on a claim must also be assessed: Are there modified or light-duty assignments available? Is the employer aware of the claimant's rights and willing to work toward getting the claimant back to work?

Case managers in workers' compensation need expertise in orthopedic injuries. Knowledge of the care providers in the geographic area can be very helpful. Common injuries, such as carpal tunnel, low back pain, and rotator cuff tears, can linger if not treated properly. The cost of inappropriate care is not just the medical benefits, which account for only about 40 percent of the claim, but the wage loss portion, which drives the price of prolonged claims for the insurance company and the employer.

Case managers also need to know how to read and evaluate rehabilitation provider records. The records should show what therapies were used, the employee's progressive ability to demonstrate increased functional capacity, and instruction by the physical therapy provider as to self-care interventions that will reinforce the office therapy. One of the areas of abuse in workers' compensation treatments has been *work hardening*. This type of therapy is supposed to simulate a modified version of the job to which the employee is expected to return. It should produce gradual progression in the functional capacity of the patient's injured area. Past abuses with these programs and a move by employers to set up light-duty programs on the job have diminished the use of work hardening programs.

Claimant Legal Representation

One of the confounding issues in workers' compensation claims is lawyers. As a rule of thumb, when there are legitimate reasons for the claimant to have legal representation, the lawyer is cooperative with case management activities. When there are hidden agendas, including the attorney's agenda to increase the costs of the claim (because he or she gets a percentage of the payout in some states), there is little cooperation with, or direct obstruction of, case management attempts. The case manager's task in these cases is to document the reasonableness of case management involvement, the goals of the case, and untoward consequences to the claimant if case management is obstructed. This documentation should be shared with the lawyer, the claimant, and the adjuster, and may be important at a later date when a hearing is due before an administrative law judge or other arbitrator. This tactic may motivate the lawyer and claimant to be more reasonable.

There are legitimate reasons for involvement of attorneys in workers' compensation claims: for example, negligence that caused the employee's injury by equipment that the employee was using when he or she was injured. In this case, the employer should move to eliminate the risk to other employees as well as join with the employee to subrogate the cost of the claim to the negligence of the equipment manufacturer.

The restriction of employee remedy for injury on the job to workers' compensation statutes has other exceptions: for example, if the employer knows that the conditions are unsafe and may lead to illness or injury. If the employer fails to warn the employees of the danger and report the conditions as required by law or does not take steps to limit the exposure to injury (for example, with respect to exposures to noxious chemicals), the employer is considered to have caused an intentional tort against an employee, one not arising out of the course of employment. This can lead to "dual injury"—the injury as a result of the exposure and the aggravation of the injury that results from the employer's conduct. Another cause for a lawyer's involvement in a workers' compensation claim is medical malpractice. Again, the employer is not liable for the physician's activities, unless the physician is an employee of the company and it can be shown that he or she was negligently treating the worker.[6]

Long-Term Disability Insurance

Long-term disability insurance plans have their own rehabilitation nurses or contract out services to private rehabilitation companies or independent case management companies. Usually the case manager in these cases will review the file and visit the claimant after a certain time threshold, which is set by the insurance company, has been passed. Often the situation will require the case manager to interview the claimant in his or her home to establish the level of his or her continuing disability and the issues that may be germane to returning the claimant to the workplace.

Long-term disability plans insure those who are disabled from their own occupation or any occupation. Those who have HIS-OCC ("his occupation") coverage (for disability from their own occupation) can usually collect up to two-thirds of their salary minus what is collected from Social Security Disability Insurance (SSDI).

HIS-OCC coverage usually lasts for two to five years; then a review is triggered to find out if the claimant can go back to work in any occupation. At this time, a medical or disability review may be done. This involves interviewing the claimant, gathering data from the claimant's physician, doing an IME if necessary, doing a transferable skills assessment, and offering training so that the claimant can engage in gainful employment.

Case managers must be able to determine if the claimant has the motivation and transferable skills that, with some training and/or adaptive equipment, will enable him or her to return to work.

Occupational Health Nursing

The worksite can be a very efficient "community of solution" to companies that wish to manage their medical, disability, and workers' compensation costs. Properly positioned and supported, occupational health nurses engage in

- health promotion, prevention of illness and injury
- early intervention with worksite injuries
- case management strategies regarding the use of the most appropriate providers, the screening of providers and claims for appropriateness of care, and coordination of care among providers.[7]

At Honeywell, the company upgraded the position of the company nurse to that of health services advisor (HSA)—in effect, a case manager over the employee/family member's continuum of care. In addition to the above responsibilities, HSAs took on advocacy roles to help employees understand and use their health insurance plan. They also helped monitor the compliance of providers and insurance companies with expected standards of care. Additionally, Honeywell used the input of HSAs to improve the design of health benefit plans, specifically to include more preventative services. Computerized record keeping was initiated to gain a better understanding of employee injury and claims patterns. This has enabled Honeywell to design preventative programs in conjunction with safety, industrial hygiene, and occupational medicine departments in the corporation. Honeywell's HSA nurses documented a 3:1 return on investment for their case management activities on selected cases.[8]

Occupational health nurses and others engaged in workers' compensation or risk management activities at the worksite should be aware of common elements of successful employer disability programs:

1. management commitment
2. safety/prevention program
3. training, involvement of employees at all levels
4. union participation
5. coordination of all departments
6. systematic procedures for use of health and rehabilitation procedures
7. early intervention/monitoring
8. accountability encouraged by rigging incentives
9. organized return-to-work policies, including light duty
10. management information system monitoring of incidents, benefits use, provider services, costs, and outcomes[9]

The responsibilities of the various parties in an integrated disability management program are as follows:

- Injured/disabled employee's responsiblity
  1. Inform company that he or she considers the experience to be work related.
  2. Produce proof of disability.
- Company's responsibility (as carried out by occupational nurse manager)
  1. Have company health professional evaluate the employee's illness or injury and provide (1) written assessment to the treating physician at the first visit and (2) a brief job description and accommodations that can be made to facilitate early return to work.
  2. Design alternative work/job to accommodate rehabilitation.

- Treating physician's responsibility
  1. Know the patient's job description and the assessment provided by the company health professional at the time of the first contact.
  2. Obtain from the patient a detailed account as to how the injury/illness occurred.
  3. Establish and communicate a return-to-work plan.
  4. Include an early return-to-work estimate as part of the initial report to the company.
  5. For long-term disability, develop protocol in the same way as for short-term, and set timetables for continued documentation.

Major Medical Indemnity Insurance

In indeminity medical insurance, large case management has been used with catastrophically ill patients when the benefit ceiling is very high and when the treatment plan may not be progressive. Typically, AIDS, cancer, and highly unusual and expensive diagnoses (e.g., Gaucher's disease, Graft vs. Host disease) are appropriate for case management because the claims representatives from the insurance side do not understand the treatments recommended and are unable to speak to accountability issues with the providers. Among the benefits of case management for these types of cases are cost containment, better coordination of benefits when there is more than one insurance carrier involved, and sorting out of subrogation issues that may be present. Carriers sometimes ask for an initial evaluation by a case manager in order to make a decision as to the cost-effectiveness of case management in the process.

Self-Funded Employer Health Insurance Plans

The Employee Retirement Income Security Act of 1974 (ERISA) created a new body of law to govern employee benefit plans. This law was enacted so that multistate employers could have plans that were not hampered by individual state regulations. It was felt that employees' rights would be protected by requiring self-funded plans to disclose a great deal more to employees concerning their rights under the plan and the fiscal health of the plan.

ERISA plans cannot be forced to comply with state-sponsored coordination of benefits (COB) rules, which mandate the order of benefit determination for covered medical expenses when more than one insurance carrier is involved. These plans must, however, be in compliance with federal statutes that may speak to benefits determination issues, especially Medicare.[10]

ERISA plans are supported by large employers and unions. The claims process may be handled by a third-party administrator or an internal claims administration process. The case manager may be internal to the company or be an agent of the third-party administrator. Most self-insured plans pay for benefits only up to a certain amount per claim. After that, they refer the claim to a reinsurance or "stop-loss" carrier that insures catastrophic claims and that may look to case management to evaluate and suggest ways to manage the case more effectively.

Some self-insured plans include their workers' compensation coverage along with health coverage. This cost containment tactic is commonly referred to as "24-hour coverage." It enables the insurance administrator to use many of the cost containment interventions that have worked so well in health insurance to contain the costs of workers' compensation. Twenty-four-hour coverage has the advantages of

- reducing administrative overhead
- avoiding duplicated payments for the same conditions billed by providers to different insurers
- minimizing the costs of litigation to determine whether an illness or injury is work related[11]

Twenty-four-hour coverage was included as part of President Clinton's Health Security Act of 1993. Title 10 of the act stipulated that a commission be set up to study how to merge health and workers' compensation coverage. The problem involves differing benefit levels, premium rates (the Clinton plan was to community-rate everyone for health coverage, but workers' compensation rates are industry and experience rated), and the question of who would regulate the combined program (states now regulate workers' compensation insurance).[12] The problem of regulation is compounded by ERISA, which has been a stumbling block to health reform legislation at the state and federal level.[13]

Reinsurance or "Stop Loss"

Self-insured companies, preferred provider organizations (PPOs), and health maintenance organizations (HMOs) all (some because of state regulation) have reinsurance policies to protect against costs incurred by catastrophically ill patients. There is usually a large deductible that is stipulated by the policy (e.g., $50,000), but the reinsurance carrier may require notification of a potential case when charges paid exceed a specified figure, such as half the insurance deductible. The stop-loss policy may also include co-pays, with the primary carrier continuing to pay 20 percent of the continuing cost outlays.[14] Some stop-loss carriers have their own case managers who get involved. They may simply have utilization review functions, may do a one-time evaluation, or may case-manage the patient over a period of time to attempt to control the cost.

Long-Term Care Insurance

Long-term care insurance is a relatively new offering of insurance companies. The policies offered are written to cover various levels of nursing care as needed by the policyholder. Depending on the provisions of the plan, skilled, intermediate, and custodial nursing care are covered. The intent is to supplement government entitlements (Medicare/Medicaid), and eligibility for benefits depends on "gatekeeper" (need or eligibility-for-care) clauses. Generally the claimant is qualified for benefits if his or her doctor orders care, but the insurance company confirms the need for services and the benefits coverage. Many policies cover home care if the claimant is unable to perform activities of daily living, and they determine the needs of the claimant and contract with a provider to perform the service.[15]

One company that works with long-term care insurance carriers is LifePlans. Its case managers perform risk management functions, determining the level of care needed and the monetary exposure of the insurance company to perform needed services. They then contract with provider organizations to perform the needed services. These services can range, depending on policy provisions and the needs of the claimant, from home care with activities of daily living to rehabilitation services and skilled inpatient care. They contract with private geriatric case managers, home care agencies, visiting nurse associations, and so on, depending on the needs of the patient and the quality of the service provider. All providers must agree to adhere to the quality standards of the referral source, The Family Caring Network, which is a subsidiary of LifePlans. The company has over 900 service providers and 2,000 care managers under contract.[16]

Private Geriatric Case Management

Private geriatric case managers are usually social workers who are hired by the family or the estate trustee of someone who is institutionalized or otherwise needs assistance with ensuring that his or her medical and social needs are being accommodated. The National Association of Private Geriatric Case Managers[17] (NAPGCM) has standards and practice guidelines that promote "humane and dignified social, psychological and health care for the elderly and their families through counseling, treatment and delivery of services by qualified, certified providers." NAPGCM defines a geriatric case manager who is qualified for full membership as one who has an advanced degree in social work, psychology, or gerontology, or a substantial equivalent (a registered nurse) who is licensed or certified in his or her state to practice independently and who has two years of supervised experience in gerontology following his or her advanced degree.[18]

Medical-Legal Consulting

Case managers may be employed by attorneys for tasks similar to those that they perform for insurance companies. Case managers get involved in personal injury, malpractice, or product liability claims. They review records, organize the medical file, arrange for expert witness exams, sort out causality issues, develop life care plans (see example in Chapter 4), and give expert testimony concerning the case.[19]

Behavioral Health Case Management

Behavioral health care is generally thought to be treatment for psychiatric problems or substance abuse. There has been tremendous growth in managed-care behavioral health as a cost containment mechanism to stem the dollar amounts spent on provision of services for these conditions. Most behavioral health case management tends to be by telephone, with the claimant gaining access to the system through an employee assistance plan (EAP). The EAP case manager determines the eligibility of the claimant for services and directs him or her to an appropriate level of services. If the claimant is incapacitated, the treatment provider or family may interact with the case manager. Behavioral health case management is practiced by social workers, nurses, certified addiction counselors (CACs), and those trained by the behavioral health company, who may or may not have advanced degrees or appropriate training.

Other Types of External Case Management

Social service professionals are charged with case management activities in selected or at-risk populations, as defined by payer sources and state and local practices. Free-standing social service agencies, special unit agencies such as area agencies on aging, and developmental disabilities units of state agencies do case management with individuals, supporting their ability to live relatively independently. Sometimes special units in planning agencies take on case management functions so as to screen, coordinate, refer, and monitor clients with special needs.[20] Knowledge of local programs and awareness of programs for which clients or claimants may be eligible may assist case managers to tap into service sources that can stretch benefit dollars or partially fund services to a client with preexisting conditions that may have been partially responsible for the illness or injury.

INTERNAL CASE MANAGEMENT

Internal case managers, or "within-the-walls" case managers, can be defined by their relationship to the institution or provider organization.

Lyon's review of case management (which failed to mention insurance or private rehabilitation case management) pointed out that many nurses and other health professionals are confused about how case management compares with nursing care delivery systems. Lyon asserted that direct patient care delivery in acute care systems does not fit the definition of *case management*, but is rather utilization review.[21] Internal case managers, then, often have an overriding utilization management function: they may choose who will be case managed, usually on the basis of diagnosis: track the patient, using critical path guidelines; interact with the treatment team regarding progress and deviations from the expected progress; and interact with the payers. Whatever the internal setting, these case managers need

- strong support from executive administration (as they may not fit into traditional hierarchical structures or may be seen as invading others' turf)

- timely and consistent information regarding patient progress, so as to track variance and inform external utilization management personnel
- unquestioned clinical expertise regarding the types of cases they cover
- skills in communication, collaboration, negotiation, family interaction, conflict resolution, and flexible response to changes in conditions and competing priorities

Internal case management should be supported as part of a unified patient services effort that combines the departments of quality assurance, utilization review, risk management, licensure/accreditation, policies and procedures, and infection control, much as Russell Coile proposed for his "outcomes management department."[22]

Acute Care

Hospitals have begun to do internal case management using various models with varying degrees of success. The case manager in the acute care setting would most likely be following a patient using a critical-path type of guide (also called a clinical algorithm, a protocol, a CareMAP, or a multidisciplinary action plan). Case management in hospitals was another outgrowth of diagnosis-related groups (DRGs) in 1983.[23] The two best known and successful models of internal case management to emerge were the New England Medical Center model and the Carondelet St. Mary's model.[24] The literature on case management coming out of the Center for Case Management in South Natick, Massachusetts, is a significant contribution to the evolution and possibilities of nursing practice.[25]

Zander distinguished the use of clinical pathways from the role of the case manager and of the case management program.[26] Case management is not a nursing care delivery system but a way of focusing accountability on an individual or group for coordinating a patient's care while ensuring preset clinical, quality, and cost outcomes. The role involves procuring, negotiating, and coordinating services and resources needed at key points or at significant variances and addressing patterns of aggregate variances. The case manager can be a direct caregiver or have a hands-off role.

Case management is used on various diagnoses, usually with the aid of a formalized critical path. Critical paths should be constructed for high-volume, expensive, or complex processes. By saving on variations of clinical outcomes, case management has been shown to reduce lengths of stay and resource utilization.

The Importance of Cultural Assessment

Cunningham and Koen asserted that a redesign of care delivery that initiates case management should include a cultural assessment of the institution as the number one (and most overlooked) task.[27] The organizational culture of the hospital must be ready, and the leadership, medical staff, and other employees must be ready for the change.

One of the biggest factors in obstructing hospital case management programs has been physicians. Many see case management as a threat to their autonomy or as a power play by the nursing department. Zander stated that obstruction by physicians can be handled and that once case management is instituted, many physicians are pleased to find that their patients get more attention. Case management demands a move to a collaborative practice model within institutions.[28] The failure of some hospitals to make case management pay may have something to do with giving up control and pinpointing accountability.

Case Management and Patient-Focused Care

Reduced lengths of stay and closer attention to resource utilization are generally supported by the effort of hospitals to move to a patient-focused care model. This care model, as advocated by Lathrop,[29] sets behavioral goals similar to those of case management programs: increased collaboration among professionals, an increase in the continuity of care, cross-training of staff regarding the skills they bring to the bedside, and empowering of staff to be more responsive to patient needs. Value-added services to patients also encompass the cognitive dimension of patient care: comforting, counseling, and educating patients and their families.

Internal case management supports the patient-focused paradigm. With the aid of charting by exception (as with CareMAPs), organizational structures that encourage all team members to follow agreed-upon guidelines for agreed-upon reasons, and continual rethinking of how the systems are working at the individual patient level, acute care systems can adapt to thrive in the post-fee-for-service age. This effort can produce improvements on a day-to-day level if these are reported for individual patients. There is then a diminished need for year-end reports or aggregate data months after reporting periods have ended. Case management programs should be expected to focus on high-volume and problem patients and continually improve the perceived delivery of care and functional health of the patient.

Requirements for Hospital Case Managers

The baseline performance requirements of a hospital case manager should be congruent with the case management program and the mission of the institution. Not every case manager has to have a specific skill set; in fact, it is better if there is a mix among a diverse group of nurses. Clinical skills, writing and oral communication skills, and negotiation skills should be expected, but case managers who have any one of the following areas of expertise can add to the effectiveness of the case management program:

- specialty clinical skills (cardiology, oncology, newborn, pediatric, asthma, brain and spinal cord injury, pulmonary disease, orthopedics, AIDS, chronic renal failure, drug and alcohol, gerontology, psychiatric, etc.)
- utilization review experience
- discharge-planning experience
- quality assurance/improvement
- infectious disease
- workers' compensation insurance programs
- home health experience
- gathering and analyzing health research
- library/computer search skills
- computer skills
- teaching skills

The members of the case management team should have complementary skills and personalities so as to enhance collaboration with each other, with patients, and with physicians and other providers.

Sampson argued that nurses are quick to embrace the collaborative interdisciplinary approach that balances both cost and quality.[30] A review of case management literature focusing on the effectiveness of case management activity indicates that the nurse is the crucial determinant of successful case management program.[31] The broader based expertise demanded by medical and psychosocial evaluations points to the need for registered nurses to assume this role rather than social workers. A community hospital could function very well with B.S.N.s who have experience with the type of patient they are following.

Sicker patients, such as those in tertiary care facilities, should be case managed by the clinical specialists. Clinical nurse specialists, or "clin-specs," are master's-prepared nurses with an expertise in a particular clinical area. They would have the technical expertise to challenge resident physicians and others whose active cooperation is required in order to keep things moving forward. The socialization of individual clin-specs to this role is another matter. Case managers need to have the "people skills" to negotiate and coach treatment teams, patients, and families. They should understand fiscal management, identification and collection of variance reports, and the clinical and health outcomes measures used in their specialty. It is a special and demanding role. Productivity and intensiveness of service determine how many patients an internal (non-clinical or hands-off) case manager can follow. For surgical patients who have fairly predictable treatment paths, a caseload of 20 patients is thought to be manageable on most surgical units. Medical patients, because they are older and needier, need one case manager for every 15 to 18 patients. Patients with the following conditions would be selected for consideration for case management at Beth Israel Medical Center in New York:

- complicated medical plan
- age over 75
- potential for falls
- potential for skin breakdown
- discharge placement problem
- noncompliance with treatment[32]

Transition to the New Paradigm

Many hospitals have their utilization review and discharge planners now trying to perform some case management functions without the training or support to do so. These nurses (and sometimes social workers) are busy trying to answer individual inquiries from external utilization management nurses and case managers. When the work is done piece-meal, it is an overwhelming and frustrating task for both the hospital nurses and the insurance company. For the hospital, it leads to payment denials; for the insurance company, it leads to unsatisfied subscribers.

Instead of having outlier patients handled by a number of nurses after they have already exceeded length-of-stay parameters, a case management program would identify probable outliers by system, disease, and patient-inherent risk factors so as to monitor and manage their care most efficiently. A case manager who knows an individual patient can alert the insurance company/HMO to the likelihood of a problem before it happens, thus opening a dialogue and widening the length-of-stay parameters and perhaps the treatment choices, where applicable.

As all services rendered by hospitals become cost centers under capitated systems, some acute care hospitals will delay or disable their case management systems until it becomes absolutely necessary for them to change.

One of the biggest near-term issues is to begin to please external case managers from insurance or HMO payers. The common fiscal and quality goals must be worked out by providers and payers with case management as one of the tools. These goals include

- length-of-stay reduction
- cost-per-case reduction
- increased patient satisfaction
- increased physician satisfaction
- increased employee satisfaction
- decreased admission/readmission rates[33]

The model, organizational design, use of incentives, and information systems wait for the cultural and goal issues to be resolved before they come in to play. The case management program is a step-by-step, bottom-up and top-down initiative that, like any QI project, needs a project manager and facilitator to make it happen.

New Markets in Case Management

As the need for nurses in hospitals dwindles and the need for nurses in home care explodes, case management programs are being marketed for a variety of settings (see Table 2–1), and learning organizations are moving to retrain hospital nurses to follow up on certain subsets of patients in "hospital-without-walls" programs, such as the Carondelet St. Mary's model. As described by Etheridge and Lamb,[34] such programs give the professional nurse case manager approximately 10 acute care and 40 community-based patients to follow at any given time. This case manager has another 40 to 50 patients who may need monthly phone contact or some minor evaluation. Risk factors triggering referral to case management are age, age of the family caregiver, number and frequency of previous admissions, and potential for complications because of multiple health or social problems.

Assessment of the patient involves the full spectrum of biopsychosocial issues that may affect the patient's health. The discharge plan is started as the patient enters the hospital, and mutually negotiated interventions are provided as problems arise. Problem groups or populations of patients are targeted and referred to the Nursing Network, which attempts to integrate care across the continuum by permitting nurses to work within the acute care setting and in the community. The high-risk patients referred include

Table 2–1 New Markets in Case Management

Potential Customer	Needs/Expectations	Case Management Product
Managed care for an HMO that integrates both acute and long-term care in a capitated, prepayment system for Medicare beneficiaries	Reduce risk of nursing home placement for the frail elderly. Decrease hospitalization and utilization of services. Promote independence at home.	Provide long-term care through the case management Medicare benefit, with supplemental services authorized by the HMO that will prevent exacerbation of illness and utilization of inpatient services.
Hospitals	Decrease LOS/decrease financial penalties from third-party payers. Generate new sources of income in the outpatient arena. Stabilize patient referral base. Capture patient/family as a lifetime customer. Diversify services by providing a community outreach program. Improve image in the community. Encourage use of inpatient services that can be used in the outpatient area (e.g., laboratory service, pharmacy). Emphasize medical staff development and satisfaction. Package inpatient and outpatient services to create product lines that can then be offered to third-party payers.	Provide a comprehensive range of programs that can be vertically integrated within the inpatient setting to decrease LOS. Consultation by a clinical nurse specialist who can provide assistance in managing populations at risk for overutilization of inpatient services. Hospital-based home care agencies will facilitate continuity of care and keep the patient within the system. Provide the hospital with the ability to extend services into the community. Influence physician practice patterns through the agency's marketing efforts. Prevent unnecessary hospital readmissions.
Employers	Reduce employee absenteeism. Reduce the risk of disability.	Evaluate health risks pertaining to an employer's workforce and provide consultation in developing programs designed to reduce risks. Provide home care for family members so the employee can continue working.
Ambulatory surgery centers	Preadmission screening, evaluation, and preoperative teaching. Postoperative follow-up.	Design protocols for specific procedures to include those services that can be provided in the home. These services can be offered to ambulatory care centers for a set fee.

continues

Table 2–1 continued

Potential Customer	Needs/Expectations	Case Management Product
Retirement centers	Prevent nursing home placement. Health care delivery on site would be a way of attracting residents. Availability of physicians to make house calls.	Offer a wellness program for the elderly. To prevent the exacerbation of illness, promote compliance and admission to an inpatient setting. Individual case management for residents who are at risk for nursing home placement. Facilitate physician home visits.
Physician group practices	Shift to outpatient arena. Diversify services to capture a larger patient population. Provide comprehensive, multidisciplinary care without incurring additional overhead expenses. Manage chronic illness in the community. Enhance patient satisfaction.	Provide a full range of services to the physician practices in the community setting. Facilitate physician productivity by decreasing the amount of time spent managing chronic illness with the benefits of case management.

Source: Reprinted from Sampson, E., The Emergence of Case Management Models, in *Outpatient Case Management: Strategies for a New Reality* by M.R. Donovan and T.A. Matson, eds., p. 91, with permission of the American Hospital Association © 1994.

- acutely ill patients in hospitals who require complex care in transitional facilities or at home
- chronically ill patients who require ambulatory care or home care services in order to prevent acute episodes
- terminally ill patients in hospices
- high-risk patients who require ambulatory care services and monitoring

Community-based clinics called *nursing wellness centers* are staffed by nurse practitioners and tend to preventative practices with risk populations, such as health promotion, screening and counseling. The Carondelet St. Mary's approach has found that community-based care nursing case managers cut costs at the *beginning* of the hospital stay because patients are not as sick and do not have to stay as long. If patients are terminally ill, there is an appropriate disposition or decision for care level that happens sooner. Acute care nurse case managers cut costs at the *end* of the hospital stay by decreasing length of stay in the hospital.[35]

One issue that has hampered the growth of case management is that often case management uses many more resources because of the case-finding activity (i.e., finding more things wrong and bringing more resources to bear), especially by social workers in social service agencies. However, case management in a hospital setting among the frail elderly has been shown to increase the ratio of reimbursement and decrease the length of stay by two days without increasing the cost per patient day in a hospital setting.[36] Handling risk populations as a revenue center using a case management model builds important components of a continuum of care. Further, clinical algorithms and case management deter inappropriate and invasive interventions, which are a chief cause of cascade iatrogenesis among the frail elderly.

Subacute Care

Subacute care is a new development that has seen phenomenal growth in the last several years. Placement of patients in subacute centers is appropriate when the patient still requires intensive nursing and/or general rehab services but does not require close medical management or frequent diagnostic testing. The payers have shifted patients into subacute care to save $300 to $700 per day.

One of the forces that created subacute care was the prospective payment initiative in 1983 using DRGs to reimburse for care. Those patients who required additional skilled nursing care were shifted to subacute settings, and Medicare picked up the reimbursement for 100 days on a cost-plus basis.

Subacute care is seen as filling a treatment gap between acute care and long-term care. The Joint Commission on Accreditation of Healthcare Organizations (Joint Commission) estimated that more than 10 percent of the daily census of 650,000 patients in hospitals would be appropriate for subacute care. Both the Joint Commission and the Commission on Accreditation of Rehabilitation Facilities (CARF) have moved into a role of surveying and accrediting subacute care programs because of the lack of other standards (licensure, regulation, or specific reimbursement category) for these facilities. Currently, only 17 states have specific laws or regulations that deal with subacute care.[37] Subacute care billings are expected to grow by 50 percent annually by the end of the decade to an estimated $10 billion per year.[38]

Subacute patients generally fall into four categories, based on intensiveness of service and length of stay:

1. *Transitional subacute*: length of stay 3 to 30 days, five to eight hours of intensive nursing and/or rehabilitation services per day. These pa-

tients are often very sick and need wound care, IV antibiotics, chemotherapy, and/or other complex care rendered by nurses. They may
need fairly heavy pharmacy or lab support. These patients are appropriate for a hospital-based nursing facility (HBNF). The difference
between the hospital and the HBNF is that in the HBNF the patient
has a set treatment plan and does not require much in the way of
diagnostics or medical decision making. These patients can do well
with a skilled team of nurses and limited intervention by physicians.
When the patient has been in the hospital for an extended period of
time, attending to mental health needs may be the first order of
business.

2. *General subacute*: length of stay 10 to 40 days, three to five hours of
   care per day. These patients tend to be elderly and need stroke or
   limb rehabilitation. The subacute care can be given in a nursing home
   with proper staffing, supervision, and support.

3. *Chronic subacute*: length of stay 60 to 90 days, three to five hours of
   care per day. This category fits those with conditions that are debilitating and require intensive services but that are also fairly stable,
   such as ventilator dependency, or cognitive impairment associated
   with a postsurgical or medical condition (e.g., Alzheimer's disease
   with hip replacement).

4. *Long-term transitional subacute*: length of stay 25 days or more, six to
   nine hours of care per day. Patients requiring intensive nursing and
   rehab services, such as medically and developmentally impaired
   pediatric patients, and patients with brain injuries, fall into this
   category. The likely outcome is long-term care placement.

Subacute care programs, like rehabilitation facilities, may use case
managers to market services, screen patients for appropriateness of admission, and match what services would be best provided. Case managers
may also be involved in negotiating fees for the care of individual patients
and updating payer sources, including payer case managers, on the progress
and expected outcomes of patients they oversee.

Case managers in subacute care need to be sensitive to consumer
confusion regarding the level of treatment and role of the facility. Families
have difficulty adjusting to the fact that the patient may not be seen every
day by the doctor and that tests or other diagnostic activities that go on in
hospitals do not take place in a subacute care facility. Finally, families and
patients are often afraid that they may not be discharged to home—that the
patient may be being set up for final disposition to the nursing home
portion of the facility. These important issues need to be addressed directly so as to limit misunderstandings.

Joint Commission accreditation regulations are drawn from existing long-term care and acute care survey requirements. The emphasis is on interdisciplinary teamwork, which implies the training and support to handle specific types of patients. Subacute programs located in skilled nursing facilities are required to employ a Minimum Data Set for Nursing Home Resident Assessment and Care (MDS) assessment and the Resident Assessment Instrument (RAI) in order to document the nature of the physical impairments so as to justify the care plan and potential for rehabilitation.

Long-Term/Nursing Home Care

As options open in noninstitutional geriatric and long-term care, and as states attempt to reduce their Medicaid expenditures, approximately 50 percent of which go to nursing homes for long-term care of elderly patients who have exhausted their financial resources, long-term care facilities are being forced to reassess their operations and customers. Some are opting to open some beds to specialized rehabilitation services (e.g., for spinal-cord-injured, brain-injured, or Alzheimer's patients), to offer subacute care, or to do outreach to the community with senior day care. One option is to improve the care process and efficiency of the facility by moving to a case management model.

The standard of care, intensiveness of services, and documentation of care are being set by RAI, the MDS, and the Resident Assessment Protocols (RAP). These instruments were introduced by the Health Care Financing Adminstration to comply with the 1987 Omnibus Budget Reconciliation Act (OBRA) mandate to improve the care of nursing home residents.

The MDS must be performed by the 14th day of admission and may be revised up until the 21st day of residency. Quarterly reviews are done of selected MDS items, and reassessments are done if the resident is admitted to the hospital or if a significant change in his or her health status occurs. Annual reassessments are done. The RAPs are done on the same schedule. These assessments are meant to indicate the areas that need to be addressed in the care plan and to document the care that is delivered.[39]

Many nursing homes continue to define their staff along functional lines: the director of nursing, the assistant director, the shift supervisor, charge nurses, treatment nurses, and nursing assistants. There is an assessment nurse to do the MDS and a care plan nurse to write the care plan following the assessment. This system has evolved due to historical reasons. The MDS was seen as a very difficult task because nurses did not entirely understand the process or reasoning behind it. The result has been fragmentation of care within the facilities because no one individual has been accountable for the care of any particular patient. Nursing home care plans are typically sketchy, with little attempt to change the plan as patient status changes and little documentation regarding progress or response to the plan of care.

Coupled with the above is the questionable quality of care given by physicians. The care tends to be reactive rather than proactive. Treatments are a response to falls or other events instead of being preventative. Physical and chemical restraints and inappropriate use of hypnotics and other drugs continue to be a problem. The MDS/RAP was instituted so as to raise the functional status and quality of life of nursing home residents. Physician treatment plans and progress notes are often still incongruent with this goal.

Case management can have a profound effect on the quality of care services, the documentation of that care, the quality of life of individual residents, and the team functioning of the staff itself. By assigning case managers to individual patients and making them responsible for doing the MDS, drawing up the care plan, following through on the documentation, checking progress with treatments, and communicating with various in-house and external providers to improve the coordination of care, nursing homes can reduce the "hassle factors" of the nursing staff and nursing administration (especially the day supervisor).

As in any group of patients, a small number of nursing home residents are typically responsible for much of the staff time. Whether these patients are wanderers, have behavioral problems, or are bedridden is not the point. A professional nurse functioning as a case manager takes on the accountability for ensuring that the treatment plan is appropriate and progressive. The few individuals who are absorbing the majority of the staff time need someone who will direct their care. Since their problems are most often not medical but behavioral, the nurse case manager has the best training and position to create a plan to deal with them. If the interventions are failing, then the documentation needs to reflect that, and steps need to be taken to address these issues. Much of the frustration felt by the nursing staff, especially the nursing assistants who are faced with the day-to-day negative effect of poor treatment plans, is due to problems with residents for which no one is willing to take responsibility.

Case management, then, makes individual nurses accountable for assessment, planning, quality improvement, infection control, communication, and documentation regarding the care delivered. A team of case managers who are not seen as line supervisors can intervene in care issues without their efforts being seen as threatening by the nonprofessional (nursing assistant) staff. The efforts of the professional nursing staff are focused not on institutional tasks (pouring medication, a.m. and p.m. care, setting up meals and feeding, etc.), but on the patient. This is the ultimate strength of a case management program in a long-term care facility.

As the life expectancy of the elderly increases, and as the expectations of society concerning the quality of care in every sector of the health care market go up, nursing homes are hard pressed to give more for less. Some are looking to subacute care revenue to offset losses incurred in taking care of Medicaid residents. All are aware of the need to build a nursing infrastructure to provide a more sophisticated level of care. Case managers can help to build the skill level and team functioning so that these sicker patients can be handled without straining the personnel and financial resources of the facility.

As with any effort to introduce case management, the program needs to be built around quality improvement principles, identifying the position requirements at the individual facility. Some role blurring occurs between nursing and social work regarding communication with the family, outside providers, and others. The nurse case manager should be interacting with them on medical issues, and the social workers can address other issues. This eliminates the problem of hospital discharge planners who give social workers inaccurate or incomplete information on the status of patients to be admitted to the facility.

Job functions within long-term care facilities need to be rewritten so as to promote teamwork. (See the sample job description/performance appraisals for nurse case managers, charge nurses and nursing assistants in Appendix 5–A.)

Rehabilitation Hospital Care

Rehabilitation hospitals have been using case managers for a number of years to coordinate the admission of a patient to a facility and interact with the external case manager, the insurance company, and the family. Some facilities use critical paths for certain diagnoses, and the role of the case manager in actually managing the case and coordinating the team will vary with the facility itself. Here again, the case manager is usually a nurse but may be a social worker or someone who is trained internally. Most successful internal case managers have the ability to speak the language of the payer. In most cases, the payer representative is a rehab RN who is an agent for the insurance carrier.

Rehab facility case managers may also have dual-function roles in that they travel to acute care facilities to see patients and meet families. Here they have a marketing function, in that they represent and assist in negotiating treatment plans and contracted charges for patients as they enter the rehab facility. Many rehab hospitals also use their case managers to offer continuing education presentations at the facility for other case managers, so as to familiarize external case managers with the services of a facility and with individuals with whom they may have only had telephone contact.

The most likely internal case manager in many facilities is the certified rehabilitation nurse, or CRRN, who is certified by the Association of Rehabilitation Nurses (ARN). Familiarity with outcomes measures, especially with the Functional Independence Measures (FIM) and its implications regarding the care needs of each patient (see Chapter 6), should also be an expectation. The rehabilitation philosophy of encouraging patient/family self-responsibility, minimizing disability via a variety of adaptive techniques, and training the family in a supportive role is something that the rehab community can teach the rest of the health delivery community.

Home Care

Since there has been such a rush to get patients out of the acute care setting into the home, home care has seen tremendous growth in the numbers and acuity levels of patients. This has led to more fragmentation of care for individuals who were discharged from the hospital before they, or their families, were functionally able to care for themselves. Specialty home care ("niche") providers have sprung up that deal with IV home care, ventilatory care, neonatal care, and "carved-out" services such as those for hemophiliacs and kidney failure patients.

Home care has also been driven by the growth in numbers of elderly Medicare patients. Due to federal cost-plus reimbursement rules, there has been little incentive for the nonprofit visiting nursing associations (VNAs) or other Medicare providers to be efficient or to control the costs of service delivery. The 1965 law establishing Medicare and Medicaid had another profound effect on home care. It shifted the scope and authority of home care services away from nursing to make physicians the gatekeepers of home care. A medical diagnosis rather than social service needs was required for home care to be given and reimbursed. Acute care needs were attended to, but the chronic care requirements of patients were ignored.[40] The VNAs and individual nurses continued to attempt to provide services that were needed but not necessarily paid for. This has driven up the cost of care.

Medicare rules that have evolved to attempt to contain the costs have resulted in burdensome paperwork, which has driven up the cost and complexity of the nursing systems without improving the quality. The Health Care Financing Administration, which is charged with ensuring the proper administration of the Medicare health benefits, has been talking about converting to prospective payment for a number of years but has not gotten beyond the stage of demonstration projects.

Many home care agencies have adopted some of the lingo of case managers but do less case management than case coordination, which they have always done. Case management does have utilization management functions, and home care case managers need to be able to demonstrate that their outcomes are cost-effective in terms of home services, not just as compared to hospital or institutional services.

There is some doubt as to the real cost-efficiency of home care. Home care may only be more cost-effective when the patient's family can help provide care.[41] Some money may be saved only because it is coming out of someone else's pocket. Increasing access to home care is driving the cost of services and placing more burdens on the system, which is attempting to take on sicker patients. Equipping, training, and supporting high-technology and specialized home care interventions require a more sophisticated infrastructure, with better information systems and tracking for outcomes measures and quality assurance. The problem is that home care has traditionally been undermanaged in terms of client assessment, worker supervision, and quality assurance.[42]

Another problem with home care services is access. In parts of cities where many of the poor and elderly reside, the safety of home nurses is a real issue, and nurses may be unwilling to risk exposure to injury or incident. Access to home care providers who can speak the language and understand the cultural aspects of targeted populations is also essential. As managed-care organizations attempt to emphasize home care over facility-based care, innovative thinking and programming will be required to meet access and quality-of-care needs for inner-city populations.

Home care nurses need to be trained and given incentives to take more control over the process of getting families and other supports in place. Home care nurses need to understand that their role is changing as management of the patient is configured along the continuum of care. They cannot do everything for the patient, and there are limits (especially time limits) to what can be done to optimize the health-related quality of life of the chronically medically ill.

Utilization management has affected home care companies recently via written protocols that offer, largely on the basis of diagnostic criteria, optimal recovery guidelines (ORGs) to cue payers and providers as to the array and intensiveness of services. The actuarial firm of Millman & Robertson has published home care case management guidelines for medical, surgical, and pediatric patients.[43] These guides are useful in establishing parameters for optimal recovery, but most chronic patients with assorted comorbidities do not fall into these categories. The guidelines are also available for automated systems for telephonic utilization review.

The guidelines clearly expect that home care nurses be engaged in cost containment activity. They also assume that a preprocedure case management assessment is done to identify baseline health status, new diagnoses, complicating medical conditions, and socioeconomic assets or challenges of the patient and family.[44]

Home care nurses need to do timely assessments and communication to the payers using guidelines to ensure that resource utilization by the home care agency is, in fact, covered. Since most discharge planning and first-encounter visits in home care do not meet this standard, it is difficult for home care agencies to meet the expected utilization guidelines. The cumbersome process of generating the treatment plans, filling out the 486 and 487 forms, having the physician sign them, and formulating the UB-92 forms makes timely notification and authorization of covered services in home care even more difficult.

Successful home care case management will need more timely notification of the need for services and a more accurate and complete data set with which to recognize care needs. A support system to collect information and transmit it to the physician, suppliers, billing, pharmacy, payers, and ancillary services (HHA, PT, OT, M.S.W., respiratory therapist, etc.) without undue duplication or errors is essential so that home care providers can absorb the service demands and survive.

Case management services can be billed under rules promulgated under guidelines in the section "Management and Evaluation of the Care Plan" of the Health Care Financing Administration's *Health Care Insurance Manual*.[45] Physicians bill for their case management activity (oversight of and sign-off on the care plan developed by the nurses). Skilled nursing visits for case management are also considered to be reasonable and necessary when underlying conditions or complications require a registered nurse to ensure that essential skilled and nonskilled care is achieving its purpose and when the complexity of the nonskilled care requires nursing to promote recovery and medical safety in view of the patient's overall condition. The success of home care agencies in collecting on case management services may be dependent on the policies of the fiscal intermediary, which vary from region to region.

PPOs

A preferred provider organization (PPO) is a type of managed care organization that contracts with a panel, or selected group of health care providers, to provide services for the insured group. PPOs often provide services to self-insured groups and take on little risk. Providers typically agree to provide services at a discount from the usual and customary fee. The PPO uses intense utilization management activity to discourage providers from gaming the system by making up for the discounts through greater utilization. Large case management is performed on high-dollar and selected diagnoses.

HMOs

Because HMOs link the financial and service delivery components so closely, case management can be a more effective tool to control resource utilization here than in most other case management settings.[46] HMO case managers have evolved, as in every other setting, more because of historical reasons within the individual organization than because of "best practice" rationales. Some organizations assign utilization review nurses in hospitals to follow subscriber length of stay and to facilitate discharge. Depending on the philosophy of the case management program, the nurse may only review the chart or may interact with the patient, the doctor, and other parties at the institution. Some HMO case managers use laptops and link up with the HMO to send and receive information. Some HMOs use telephonic utilization review nurses to promote early discharge to the most appropriate setting.

Some HMOs have certain diagnoses and catastrophically ill patients followed by case managers throughout the trajectory or "arc" of care that begins when the patient is identified as high risk, proceeds through the treatment processes and an array of service providers, and, it is hoped, ends when the patient is at home on the path to full recovery. Since most sickness eventually becomes disease and most disease becomes chronic illness, the abilities of these case managers to teach, coordinate, negotiate, and coach patients and their families become critical to the success of the case management unit that is charged with modulating resource use.

HMOs have demonstrated success in improving the quality of care while moderating the cost compared to fee-for-service medicine.[47] HMO medical practice is moving rapidly from experience-based to evidence-based medicine.[48] What this means in a practical sense is that the physicians have been given incentives to follow clinical algorithms or critical pathways for selected diagnoses and that this has effected improvement in the medical outcome. Physicians are doing less individual decision making on the basis of their experience or their gut feeling, and the outcome for most patients is better. This change in practice makes the physician's role more collaborative, that of a "guide on the side" rather than a "sage on the stage."[49]

Nurse Case Managers and Primary Care Physicians

Primary care physicians/providers (PCPs) in group-model HMOs are employees of the organization and thus can easily be trained and supported to follow certain protocols to ensure care quality and cost control. Individual-practice-association-model HMOs rely on capitation, or a per-member-per-month (PMPM) fee, to pay PCPs for the care they render to subscribers. Usually only a portion of the PMPM payment is sent. The rest is held in a risk pool of money that will pay for unexpected utilization of resources or referrals made by the PCP.

Most PCPs pride themselves as being the "case managers" of any given patient's care. However an HMO case manager can assist PCPs to control the resource use of chronic and catastrophically ill patients. When the case manager works with the PCPs to address nonmedical issues and coordinate care, the health outcome and subscriber/patient satisfaction can rise. Costs, resource use, and "daily hassles" for the PCP can go down. A smooth-running referral system and training of case managers and PCPs on how to collaborate can prevent some of the turf wars that have resulted in some HMOs.

Nurse case managers can assist PCPs in a number of ways. Besides coordinating the care of catastrophic illnesses, they can answer patient and family inquiries and address issues that may be important but not medically related. Some patients have very high and unrealistic demands for service or the eventual outcome of care. The case manager can reinforce information given by the PCP concerning the eventual outcome or the rationale for treatment choices. (See Case Study 4 in Chapter 3 for an illustration of some of these roles.)

Exhibits 2–1 and 2–2 show a case management outcomes worksheet and a focused progress report template. Each participant in the patient's care, including the patient and family, can be given one of these to fill out on a periodic basis.

Case Management and Cost Control

As previously stated, most HMOs buy reinsurance to indemnify themselves against unpredictable loss. By using case management, HMOs can keep their reinsurance rates and co-pays for coverage under control. Pacificare's Medical Group/Independent Physician Association (PMG/IPA) model HMO uses case managers to assist medical groups and inde-

Exhibit 2–1 Case Management Outcomes Worksheet

Baseline Status	Short-Term Goals	Drivers/Inhibitors	Long-Term Goals
Patient medical history or mechanism of injury	1. 2.	1. 2.	1. 2.
Diagnoses:			
Medical care plan goals: 1. 2.			

Patient health status
  physical functioning:
  role functioning:
  mental functioning:
  well-being:
  health perceptions:			

Social support inventory			
Self-stated goals:			
Family/significant other goals:			
Monetary risk exposure: $____			

Note: The case manager needs to assess the starting point, categories of goal areas, and kinds of improvements indicated. Factors that drive or motivate patients, families, and providers need to be identified, along with issues that may delay or obstruct appropriate care or meeting goals. Since case managers are also utilization managers, they need to begin the process of estimating what expenses and categories of expenses are likely to be incurred to reach the goals.

pendent physician associations to coordinate complex and costly cases without charge to the physician capitation.[50] Case managers are assigned to a geographic area or a large group practice. Referrals to case management are made from the groups themselves or may be triggered from a hospital that calls to verify eligibility of a subscriber for services. Certain ICD-9 codes may prompt case management intervention, or referrals can be made from patients, members, employers, marketing, utilization review, or the quality assurance department.

Exhibit 2–2 Outcomes-Focused Progress Notes

Problem Area	Monthly Goal	Measure of Meeting Goal (7-Point Scale)	Long-Term Goal
Medical goals		1 2 3 4 5 6 7	
Feeling states goals		1 2 3 4 5 6 7	
Functional and ADL goals		1 2 3 4 5 6 7	
Patient self-stated goals		1 2 3 4 5 6 7	
Family-stated goals		1 2 3 4 5 6 7	
Other:		1 2 3 4 5 6 7	

Additional comments:

Changes in care plan:

Pacificare's case management is on site, and is initiated by a complete review of the case, the medical record, and interviews with the treatment providers. A case management plan may include referral to community resources and not just referrals of patients within the provider network. Bower describes an HMO case management model for a group-practice HMO that stipulates clear utilization management functions as well as case management functions to the nurses, who assume 24-hour-a-day, 7-day-a-week responsibility for the patients they case-manage.[51]

Telephonic Case Management

Some HMOs use telephonic case managers almost exclusively for care direction across the continuum: to urge discharge from the hospital, arrange for subacute care, and negotiate the home care, all without seeing the patient. There is a heavy utilization management emphasis. Care is directed with the aid of information from the provider facility, the family, and occasionally the physician. It is difficult to know the efficiency or effectiveness of such programs. The training, information/decision support, and case management philosophy can vary widely. An RN from North Dakota can be case-managing an HMO patient in Newark, New Jersey. Lack of knowledge of the local health providers and miscommunication due to cultural issues are bound to cause confusion.

There is scant literature concerning the use of telephonic case management and utilization review. The practices, decision support, and philosophies of these systems are as variable as the numbers of companies engaging in this enterprise. Suffice it to say that telephonic utilization review case management is among the most vilified of all case management activities.

Utilization Review/Utilization Management

Utilization review (UR) generally applies to retrospective activities designed to flag and deny payment for services that were medically unnecessary, inappropriate (as with palliative care), ineffective, or not covered by the insurance plan. Utilization management (UM) does the same thing, but *prospectively* authorizes services and *concurrently* monitors service delivery and patient status. UR/UM tasks vary between payer and provider sources and generally have high rates of return on investment on paper, but add little value to the actual quality of care rendered or the health outcome of the patient.

Written or computerized guidelines for admission to an inpatient facility or for intensiveness of outpatient services drive decisions made by UM nurses. Payment for services rendered is often denied because of poor documentation of the need for services, poor documentation of the services link to the condition or the covered benefit, or the untimeliness of the authorization-to-treat request. There is a movement toward a uniform data set for medical documentation, but the standards process is still being worked out. The ease of information flow that is emerging through automation will demand that all providers get some high-tech capability in order to be competitive.[52]

There has been much abuse of the claims process on both the payer and provider sides of the UM street, and some case law adjudication concerning general practices in UM has emerged.

The Utilization Review Accreditation Commission (URAC) was formed in 1990 out of an initiative led by the American Managed Care and Review Association (AMCRA), a trade association of UR companies, PPOs, and HMOs, to standardize the practice of UR and prevent the regulation of UR companies, which has occurred in some states.[53] URAC specifies that UR shall collect only information necessary to certify the admission, treatment, or length of stay. URAC standards stipulate what kinds of information are to be requested for retrospective chart reviews. Procedures for review determination also stipulate that certification determinations be made within two days' receipt of necessary information on a proposed admission or service. Further standards cover procedures for review determination, documentation of the certification or denial of service, the appeals process, staff and program qualifications, accessibility of the reviewing personnel, and accessibility of records for on-site review.[54]

Medicare regulations have mandated UR by peer review organizations, (PROs). PROs are required to review hospital readmissions within 31 days of discharge, review beneficiary complaints about the quality of hospital services, and reduce quality problems, such as unavoidable deaths or unnecessary services. The American Medical Peer Review Association sets standards for the PROs and their activities.[55] (See Exhibit 2–3 on documentation rules for ambulatory encounters.)

It is probable that as more people are covered under managed-care plans and as utilization authorization requests and referrals are communicated electronically, the place of UR companies will diminish. UM functions are becoming more functions of telephonic case management in this situation.

Telephonic Triage and Help Services

Telephone triage has grown in a number of different areas of health delivery, for a number of reasons. HMOs have used nurses as gatekeepers for calls from subscribers to cut costs. Hospitals have used telephonic systems to offer assistance with health information and to increase awareness of services provided by the hospital. There are many "hot lines" operating that deal with focused health information (drug abuse, mental distress, AIDS) or are simply safety nets designed to keep tabs on the elderly or other at-risk populations. Many calls are made simply for reassurance. Since physicians do not listen closely enough, they often miss what the real intent of the call is. Most calls come from women or the elderly, and most of the problems cited are chronic in nature.[56] Telephone triage can help eliminate unnecessary office or ER visits, educate subscribers, and improve relations with the PCP and the HMO.

Some HMOs and other large managed-care entities have services that answer questions from subscribers concerning a variety of health-related issues. The idea here is to provide "demand management." Although managed-care plans try to hold costs down by limiting access or "supply" of services, the concept behind demand management is to encourage self-care and informed decision making. Informed decision making on the part of consumers should change their perception of the need to seek professional care, resulting in reduced demand for services.[57]

The use of a publicized telephonic service is designed to relieve the demand for services in the following way. Subscribers call a toll-free number with their symptoms and health problems and speak to nurses

Exhibit 2–3 Guidelines for Documentation of Ambulatory Encounters

Operational philosophy—A patient's health record should include sufficient information:
1. to assess the previous treatment,
2. to ensure continuity of care, and
3. to ensure necessary and appropriate testing and/or therapy.

Guidelines for documentation for ambulatory encounters:
1. The medical record should be clearly legible and reviewable.
2. The documentation of a patient encounter should include: clinical history, clinical findings, assessment, and plan for care.
3. The plan of care should include, when appropriate:
   - medications, including frequency and dosage;
   - specific instructions for follow-up;
   - informed consent; and
   - education, when appropriate, indicating patient participation.
4. The documentation should support that the intensity of the patient evaluation and treatment reflected the reason for the encounter, the intensity of the problem, and the findings of the examination.
5. It is suggested that the date and time of day of each encounter be documented.
6. Patient non-compliance, such as failure to return for an appointment, should be documented.
7. Significant X-rays, lab tests, and other ancillary study results should be addressed.
8. The reason for X-rays, lab tests, and other ancillary studies should be documented in the medical record.
9. The originator of the medical records entry should be identifiable.
10. If the physician assumes management of a patient in another locale, that management should be documented in the appropriate medical record.
11. Relevant risk factors should be identified.
12. When appropriate, past and present diagnoses should be accessible to the consulting/treating physician.
13. Patient referrals and consultations should be documented.
    Referral: Care transferred to another physician who assumes management of the care which precipitated the referral.
    Consultation: The primary physician retains responsibility for the patient.
14. The documentation in the record should support the CPT/ICD codes billed.

Source: Courtesy of the American Medical Peer Review Association, Washington, D.C.

trained to interview patients over the phone. They have a perceived need for services that may or may not be well founded. Ideally, the subscribers themselves are interviewed. Age, symptoms and symptom severity, personal and family health history, and the sequence of events leading to the call are ascertained. An attempt is made to judge the truthfulness of the callers' claims and their emotional state. Callers may be directed to seek care based on their degree of debilitation or on their distance from a facility or other access issue.[58]

Telephonic health services use computer-aided protocols and decision trees to assist the nurse or other counselor in supplying information concerning self-management of chronic disease or minor illness, preventive self-management (especially with perinatal care), and major diagnostic or therapeutic procedures.

The quality of service rendered by telephonic triage is dependent on the training, the effectiveness of the computer protocols and decision support, and the time allotted for each call. Time allotments may range from an expected 3 minutes per call to 30 to 45 minutes, and the nurse may also make call-back appointments to follow up with the subscriber.

NOTES

1. R. Howe, ed., *Case Management for Healthcare Professionals* (Chicago: Percept Press, 1994).

2. M.R. Donovan and T.A Matson, eds., *Outpatient Case Management: Strategies for a New Reality* (Chicago: American Hospital Publishing, 1994).

3. N. Cope and K. Hall, Head Injury Rehabilitation: Benefit of Early Intervention, *Archives of Physical Medicine and Rehabilitation* 63 (1982):433–437.

4. A.F. Southwick, *The Law of Hospital and Health Administration*, 2nd ed. (Ann Arbor, Mich.: Health Administration Press, 1988), 33–34.

5. A. Blum and R. Mauch, RN Case Manager Can Help Provide Appropriate Care, Cost Management, *Occupational Health and Safety* 59, no. 4 (1990):68–69.

6. Southwick, *Law of Hospital and Health Administration*.

7. B.J. Burgel, *Innovation at the Worksite: Delivery of Nurse Managed Primary Health Care Services* (Washington, D.C.: American Nurses Publishing, 1992).

8. J. M. Bey et al., The Nurse as Health Manager, *Business and Health*, October 1990, 24–31.

9. R. Habeck, Managing Disability in Industry, *Journal of the National Association for Health Professionals in the Private Sector* 6, no. 4 (1991):141–146.

10. T. Holloway et al., *The Coordination of Benefits Handbook* (Washington, D.C.: Thompson Publishing Group, 1995), 3–4.

11. M. Major, 24-Hour Coverage: A Concept Whose Time Has Come? *The Case Manager* 5, no. 2 (1994):62–68.

12. G. Countryman, For Workers' Comp, Say No to Reform, *New York Times*, July 30, 1994, A–20.

13. C. Petersen, State, Feds Scuffle over ERISA, *Managed Healthcare* 5, no. 1 (1994):12–14.

14. E.B. Pascuzzi, Claims and Benefits Administration, in *The Managed Healthcare Handbook*, 2nd ed., ed. P. Kongstvedt (Gaithersburg, Md.: Aspen Publishers, Inc., 1993), 227–228.

15. National Association of Insurance Commissioners, *A Shopper's Guide to Long Term Care Insurance* (Kansas City, Mo.: 1993).

16. A. Ingoldsby, personal communication to author, 1995, LifePlans/Family Caring Network, Waltham, Mass.

17. National Associaton of Private Geriatric Case Managers, 655 North Alveron Way, Suite 108, Tucson, Ariz. 85711.

18. C. Polich et al., *Managing Health Care for the Elderly* (New York: John Wiley & Sons, Inc., 1993), 102–103, 176.

19. B. Overby, Legal Consulting: The Case Manager in the Courtroom, *The Case Manager* 4, no. 1 (1993):71–75.

20. R. Applebaum and C. Austin, *Long-Term Care Case Managment* (New York: Springer Publishing Co., Inc., 1990), 46–49.

21. J.C. Lyon, Models of Nursing Care and Case Management: Clarification of Terms, *Nursing Economics* 11, no. 3 (1993):163–169.

22. R. Coile, *The New Medicine* (Gaithersburg, Md.: Aspen Publishers, Inc., 1990), 347–350.

23. K. Zander, Case Management in Acute Care: Making All the Connections, *The Case Manager* 2, no. 1 (1991): 39–43.

24. P. Etheridge and G. Lamb, Professional Nursing Case Management Improves Quality, Access and Costs, *Nursing Management* 20, no. 3 (1990):30–35.

25. *D.E.F.I.N.I.T.I.O.N.* and *The New Definition* are published quarterly by the Center for Case Management, Inc., 6 Pleasant St., South Natick, Mass. 01760. Subscriptions are free on request; there is a nominal charge for back issues. Phone (508) 651-2600.

26. K. Zander, History, Rationale, and Clarification of Acute Care Case Management (Paper presented at the meeting of the Individual Case Management Association, Orlando, Fla., September, 1993).

27. L.G. Cunningham and M.J. Koen, Acute Care Case Management: Integration for Providers and Payors, *The Case Manager* 5, no. 5 (1994): 53–60.

28. K. Zander, *History, Rationale, and Clarification of Acute Care Case Management* 1993.

29. P. Lathrop, *Restructuring Health Care* (San Francisco: Jossey-Bass, Inc. Publishers), 89ff.

30. E. Sampson, The Emergence of Case Management Models, in *Outpatient Case Management: Strategies for a New Reality*, ed. M.R. Donovan and T.A. Matson (Chicago: American Hospital Association, 1994), 85.

31. E.A. Erkel, The Impact of Case Management in Preventive Services, *Journal of Nursing Administration* 23, no. 1 (1993):27–32.

32. E.L. Cohen and T.G. Cesta, *Nursing Case Management: From Concept to Evaluation* (St. Louis, Mo.: C.V. Mosby Co., 1993), 113–114.

33. Cunningham and Koen, Acute Care Case Management, 54.

34. Ethridge and Lamb, Professional Nursing Case Management.

35. Ethridge and Lamb, Professional Nursing Case Management, 33.

36. R.S. Trella, A Multidisciplinary Approach to Case Management of Frail, Elderly Hospitalized Older Adults, *Journal of Nursing Administration* 23, no.2 (1993):20–26.

37. N. Sawyer, Subacute Care: Growing Segment in Health Care Continuum, *The Case Manager* 5, no. 4 (1994):93–103.

38. Joint Commission on Accreditation of Healthcare Organizations, *1995 Survey Protocol for Subacute Programs* (Oakbrook Terrace, Ill.: 1995), 1.

39. Health Care Financing Administration, *Long Term Care Resident Assessment Instrument Training Manual* (Washington, D.C.: 1990).

40. P. Cloonan, Managing Home Care, in *Key Aspects of Caring for the Chronically Ill*, ed. S.G. Funk et al. (New York: Springer Publishing Co., Inc., 1993), 40–41.

41. K. Anderson, Is It Still Home Sweet Home Care? *Business and Health,* January 1993, 42–46.

42. D. Gould and K.D. Haslanger, Home Care Prospects in an Era of Health Care Reform, *Journal of Ambulatory Care Management* 16, no. 4 (1993):9–19.

43. R.L. Doyle et al., *Healthcare Management Guidelines,* Vol. 4, *Home Care and Case Management* (San Diego, Calif.: Millman & Robertson, 1994).

44. Doyle, *Healthcare Management Guidelines,* 2.1.

45. Health Care Financing Administration, *Health Care Insurance Manual-11,* Revision 222 (Washington D.C.: 1989).

46. L.L. Hicks et al., *Role of the Nurse in Managed Care* (Washington, D.C.: American Nurses Association, 1993), 49.

47. L.F. Rossiter, The Research Agenda in Managed Care, in *Making Managed Care Work,* ed. P. Boland (Gaithersburg, Md.: Aspen Publishers, Inc., 1993), 582.

48. L.S. Katz, The New Medicine: Beyond Managed Care, *HMO Practice* 8, no.3 (1994):100–102.

49. B. Austine and E.H. Wagner, letter to the editor in *HMO Practice* 8, no. 4 (1994):190.

50. HMO Case Management: Medical Group Model, *The Case Manager* 3, no. 4 (1992):35–38.

51. K.A. Bower, *Case Management by Nurses* (Washington, D.C.: American Nurses Association, 1992), 40–41.

52. H. Anderson, Plugging in National Networks: Are Hospital Business Offices an Endangered Species? *Medical Claims Management* 1, no. 1 (1993):37–43.

53. M. O'Kane, Outside Accreditation of Managed Care Plans, in *The Managed Healthcare Handbook,* 2nd ed., ed. P. Kongstvedt (Gaithersburg, Md.: Aspen Publishers, Inc., 1993), 237.

54. Utilization Review Accreditation Commission, Inc., *National Utilization Review Standards* (Washington, D.C.: 1991).

55. D. Ermann, Hospital Utilization Review: Past Experience, Future Directions, *Journal of Health Politics, Policy and Law* 13 (1988):683–704.

56. S.Q. Wheeler, *Telephone Triage* (Albany, N.Y.: Delmar, 1994), 5, 8, 14.

57. C.S. Russel, personal communication to author, 1994, Health Decisions, Inc., Golden, Colo.

58. Wheeler, *Telephone Triage,* 80–85.

3

Case Studies Across the Continuum of Care

The *continuum of care* is generally defined as the patient's entire sequence of interactions with the health care system. It begins sometime before the patient's encounter with his or her doctor and before his or her decision to seek care. Defined for this book, however, the continuum of care includes the patient's self care; thus, it begins with how the patient manages his or her life and the way he or she copes with the stress of daily life.

Case management has traditionally been triggered by events, such as catastrophic injury, exceeding a dollar threshold in terms of medical claims made by providers of care, or the diagnosis of a possible catastrophic disease, such as cancer or AIDS. These triggers are only moderately effective in managing the cost or improving the patient outcome. The traditional insurance perspective is that catastrophic cases are going to be expensive whether they are case managed or not. Often, the treatment choices are limited to fixing the injuries. Case management can monitor the case and do early discharge planning to ensure that the patient moves from the acute care to rehabilitation and to home without lingering, thus making the care more efficient. With many catastrophic cases, the policy covers only up to a certain dollar figure, and although case management can stretch benefit dollars, there is no incentive for the insurance company to utilize a case manager.

Certain high-cost diagnoses may trigger case management activity, but a person's diagnosis is a poor predictor of how much money will be spent on the individual over the course of his or her disease (see Chapter 6). Dollar thresholds are not good predictors of the usefulness of case management activity because the treatment plan is already set. The case manager can often do little to influence the course of care.

The following cases are examples of intervention in the care of patients so as to optimize the health outcome of the patient as well as to save the employer or insurance company money.

CASE STUDY #1: PERINATAL CARE

Perinatal care focuses on pregnancy, newborn, and early infant child care. Although pregnancy is not a disease, one-fourth of all pregnant women are at risk for some kind of untoward event, costing an average of $20,000 per birth and early child care. Some cases of premature newborns can cost hundreds of thousands of dollars. Perinatal case managers screen mothers for potential for complications, and if certain risk factors are identified (e.g., smoking, previous preterm delivery, preterm labor this pregnancy, drug/alchohol use), the mother is followed and coached concerning behaviors and health status. This case study is also an example of *disease state management* (see Appendix B).

Case History

Annie R. is a 24-year-old black woman who has a history of three pregnancies—the first one electively aborted, the second a normal-term birth, and the third a preterm birth at 36 weeks. She shows mild gestational diabetes at 36 weeks. She also smokes one-half pack to one pack of cigarettes per day. She was seen by the perinatal nurse after seeing the gynecologist, who confirmed the pregnancy at nine weeks. The perinatal case manager is an employee of a company that specializes in these kinds of problems. The insurance company hired the agency for the sole purpose of screening for potential problem pregnancies and case-managing those women most likely to have problems.

The insurance company has "carved out" this high-risk population and contracted with experts to follow the high-risk pregnancies so as to lessen the possible complications of the pregnancy and limit the company's monetary exposure to a high-cost, premature birth.

Annie is given some forms to fill out in her doctor's office concerning her previous history. The preterm births and abortion in the past prompt the assignment of a case manager to visit Annie at her house and do an assessment that identifies other risk factors. Annie works at a retail store stocking shelves, and often must lift or manipulate boxes up to 40 pounds. Annie quit school during her junior year and has a GED certificate. She rarely reads and does not take much interest in pamphlets offered to her concerning the expected course of her pregnancy.

The nurse case manager has protocols that prompt her to see Annie three times during her pregnancy, review educational material with her, and telephone her to obtain information concerning her status and to reinforce the educational material. A smoking-cessation program is offered, and the case manager talks to Annie's common-law husband concerning the need for a stable lifestyle and the smoking cessation. With the permission of the patient, the case manager contacts Annie's supervisor at work and asks for a light-duty assignment during the pregnancy. All these actions are designed to lessen the chance of a preterm birth. A sample return on investment for the insurance company is given below.

Return on Investment for Screening and Case-Managing High-Risk Pregnancies

For each 1,000 births, 250 are preterm or have complications. These 250 cases cost the company $5,120,000 last year, or an average of $20,480 each. Use of risk assessment on all pregnant patients and the initiation of case management, education, and lifestyle changes reduce the number and severity of complications by 63 percent, leaving 157.5 patients with an average cost for perinatal care of $10,226. This cost is still higher than a normal pregnancy, but represents a cost saving per case of $10,254.

Return on investment (ROI) of case management is calculated as follows:

Cost of screening 1,000 patients at $200 per patient:	$ 200,000
Cost of case management of 250 patients at $1,200 each case:	$ 300,000
Cost of screening and case management combined:	$ 500,000
Costs of high-risk patients before the program was initiated:	$5,120,000
Dollars spent after program was initiated:	
(157.5 × $10,226) + (92.5 × $20,480) + $500,000 = $4,004,995	
Dollars saved by case management:	$1,115,005
Dollars spent on case management:	$ 500,000
Return on investment ($1,115,005/500,000):	$2.23/$1.00

In the above example, $2.23 was saved for every dollar spent to screen and case-manage high-risk pregnant women. The company may actually save more money because the children are likely to be more healthy and to require fewer medical interventions as they grow older. The employer saves on his or her experience-rated health insurance, so the premium rates can be held steady. The employee sees that the company cares about her and her family. Thus, case management brings value that can be seen in dollars spent in the present and the future and in good will.

CASE STUDY #2: TRAUMATIC HEAD INJURY

Joe D. is severely injured in his automobile while driving from one worksite to the next in his job as a civil engineer. He suffers a closed head injury and a complete L-1 spinal cord injury (SCI) and is admitted to a trauma unit. He lies in a coma on a ventilator and requires surgery to repair the injuries. Because he has a $1 million cap on the personal injury protection (PIP) coverage of his auto policy, the auto insurance company sends a case manager to the trauma unit to open the case.

Jane, the nurse case manager, meets with the wife and her family in the waiting room of the hospital. She explains her purpose in being there and begins to gather information from the family and the medical record concerning Joe's medical history, his work history, the mechanism of his injuries, and the projected treatment plan. During the course of her data collection, she discovers that Joe was officially on duty for his employer. She notifies her claims manager, who notifies the benefits coordinator of the insurance company. The benefits coordinator talks with the company and determines that since Joe was on the job, the coverage for the injury is the responsibility of the workers' compensation insurance company. The auto carrier informs the workers' comp carrier of the intent to subrogate the claim to the workers' comp carrier, and the latter sends a case manager to investigate further.

The workers' comp carrier accepts responsibility for Joe's claim and places its case manager on the case. The second case manager, Mary, gets a projection from the neurosurgeon concerning the future needs of the patient so that the insurance company can project its total cost exposure on the claim. These costs include all projected surgeries and hospitalizations, rehabilitation, adaptive equipment, wage loss, and (in some states) vocational rehabilitation.

The goal of the treatment plan for Joe is maximum medical improvement, or the highest physical functioning that can be obtained. Since the workers' comp carrier pays all the costs of the claim, it has the case manager follow the case closely so as to have the patient transferred to a rehab facility that can best treat the type of injury Joe has as early as possible. The rehab facility has an internal case manager who comes to see

Joe in the hospital and gets information concerning his condition so as to predict his treatment needs and likely level of recovery.

When Joe leaves the acute care hospital, he is admitted to the rehab facility. His projected length of stay is three months. His case is covered in a weekly team meeting attended by the physician and all members of the treatment team, including the internal case manager and the case manager from the workers' comp carrier. Treatment goals and plans are discussed. The external (workers' comp) case manager checks with the family regarding their perception of the quality of care given to Joe. She also makes an appointment with the family to see the structure of the home setting so that arrangements can be made for adapting his house for his wheelchair.

Construction on Joe's house begins so that he can be sent home. An outside ramp is installed to make the house accessible by wheelchair, and a room downstairs in the house is adapted to a bedroom. A new wheelchair-accessible bathroom is installed, with safety features that will allow Joe to do most of his hygiene himself. Joe is discharged to home with follow-up care, including cognitive remediation for deficits caused by his closed head injury.

The case manager monitors the contractor, the rehab facility, the home care agency, and the cognitive remediation specialists to ensure that the services rendered are rendered as planned and are within the projected budget. She also projects an end to treatment when there is no longer progress. Later, she projects the total costs of future care so that the company can set aside its reserves to pay for a lifetime of care needs.

CASE STUDY #3: OCCUPATIONAL HEALTH CASE MANAGEMENT

Gretel, the occupational health nurse for the Super Soup Company, has a complex job. As a master's-prepared, certified occupational health nurse, she does routine physicals on new employees, listens to and acts on employee concerns about plant safety, and, with the assistance of a secretary, keeps records for the state and federal occupational health and safety inspectors.

Gretel also is aware of some of the routine health needs of her employees. She keeps a list of those who have diabetes and encourages them to come for routine screening to ensure that their blood sugar is controlled. Gretel monitors the types of injuries that occur in the plant and follows patients who are injured to bring them back to work as soon as possible.

Mertyl is one of the workers on the packing line. She has reported an injury to her lower back. Mertyl wants to go to her chiropractor and asks if the company will pay for it. Gretel has no problem with chiropractors because she knows they are relatively low-cost providers who often assist with pain control and encourage the patient to be active and engage in self-care behaviors. Gretel directs Mertyl to an approved chiropractic provider, who provides Gretel with his diagnosis and treatment plan. He projects three weeks of visits with manipulation three times a week, two weeks of visits with manipulation twice a week, and a follow-up visit two weeks later. He cautions against Mertyl's lifting anything more than ten pounds twice per day.

Gretel talks with Mertyl's supervisor about getting a light-duty assignment. She knows that light duty will enable her to monitor Mertyl more closely without the risk of injury. An office position is found that involves sitting, standing, and walking tasks, but no lifting. Mertyl is also asked to watch safety films and a film on techniques for lifting and moving heavy boxes. As part of the program, she is asked to demonstrate her newly learned techniques to Gretel. After six weeks, Mertyl returns to her position on the assembly line.

CASE STUDY #4: MANAGEMENT OF HEART DISEASE IN AN ELDERLY WOMAN

Polly is a 72-year-old white woman with a history of rheumatic heart disease as a child. She has borne five children. The last pregnancy, when she was 39 years old, was taxing in that she was diagnosed with congestive heart failure and pneumonia. She spent the last seven weeks of her pregnancy on total bedrest.

Polly continued to complain of fatigue, shortness of breath, and swollen ankles after the birth of her last child, and in 1970 had a mitral commissurotomy done to open up her calcified mitral valve. Now the same symptoms are occurring at increasing frequency, and Polly is unable to walk a flight of stairs without marked dyspnea. She does not have fond memories of the first surgery and will not discuss replacement of the mitral valve as an option.

Polly and her husband are offered enrollment in a Medicare HMO. They see this as an opportunity to not have to pay for Medigap insurance and hope that by belonging to an HMO they will not have to worry about medical bills.

Polly's overall health continues to deteriorate. Because of her chronic congestive heart failure, blood flow through the liver is sluggish, and the liver is congested and slightly enlarged. Her liver enzymes are elevated to a point slightly above normal. She also complains of sleep apnea, which prevents her from restful sleep. This worsens her own perception of her health, and she has bouts of depression. Petechia are seen on her nose and cheeks, which betray late-stage chronic congestive failure. Her doctor has adjusted her medication a number of times without any improvement in her functioning or perception of well-being. Her children urge her to have the mitral valve replacement surgery.

Polly's daughter is a nurse, but she lives in California and feels frustrated that she cannot assist her mother to decide which is the best course of therapy to take. She suggests that her mother ask for a nurse case manager in order to help her sort out her feelings regarding surgery and to suggest who in the HMO plan would be the best doctor to perform it. The family doctor is happy to have someone to assist his patient. He is frustrated that he cannot offer her any relief for her constant complaints of shortness of breath, fatigue, and inability to get a good night's sleep.

Polly is visited by the nurse case manager, who talks with her and her husband about her medical problems. She also discovers that they live alone in a large house. Since Polly is unable to keep the house clean, she worries constantly about the house and blames herself for being unable to perform the expected role of wife and mother (even though the children are gone). Polly also suffers from the heat in the summer because she only has one air conditioner, which is placed in the bedroom. The nurse case manager recommends to Polly and her husband that it may be time for them to consider moving to an air-conditioned apartment where there are no stairs to climb. An apartment would also be easier to keep clean.

The nurse case manager reviews Polly's personal life goals with her in order to assist Polly in making a decision regarding surgery. Since Polly is now unable to perform activities that she regards as normal and essential to her daily life, she assents to surgery. Polly is referred to a facility that does over 1,000 surgeries a year, including many mitral valve replacements. A cardiac catheterization is done, which shows that the tricuspid valve is also leaking badly.

The tertiary care hospital to which Polly was referred has a clinical specialist nurse who acts as a liaison to Polly, her family, the referring physician, and the HMO case manager. The task is essentially that of an internal case manager. The services she provides help the HMO and Polly to predict and make arrangements for discharge planning so that the transition to home is facilitated.

Polly has a mitral valve replacement and an annular repair of her tricuspid valve. She goes home and does well for a time. The wound heals well, and she is able to sleep well at night for eight months after surgery. She is able to assume some of the activities she avoided before surgery and is able to see more of her grandchildren. Gradually, however, she begins to complain of lack of sleep (sleep apnea), loss of appetite, chronic fatigue, and pains in her legs that resemble cramps. Her doctor is unable to be of any assistance in diagnosing what is causing the cramping pain. Polly eventually asks to see the case manager.

About this time, Polly has an acute admission to the hospital for fatigue and shortness of breath. Her hemoglobin has dropped to 6.2 from its baseline of 9.5. Her H & H was within expected limits only 10 days prior to the admission. The reason for the blood loss is a mystery. There is no occult blood in the stool. The coumadin dose is being monitored via Protimes and International Ratios (INRs), which are in the proper range.

The hospital physicians recommend an endoscopy, and when that fails to show any reason for blood loss, a colonoscopy. This is also negative. A hematologist is asked to see Polly, and he recommends doing a bone marrow biopsy. By this time, Polly is very fatigued and discouraged. She meets with the HMO case manager and they talk about the future. Polly does not want the bone marrow biopsy. She is afraid of the pain. She is also afraid that cancer might be found and that she would be compelled to take treatments for it. She is now losing weight and complaining constantly of weakness.

The HMO case manager again assesses with Polly her personal goals. At first, Polly says she has to live because she has to take care of her husband and her children, who are now grown and married. As she talks, she realizes that her motivation to go on is diminished now compared to a year earlier. She does not like being in the hospital, but wishes she could sleep better at night.

The case manager arranges for Polly to see a pulmonologist, who recommends a trial course of treatment for the sleep apnea consisting of noninvasive positive pressure ventilation (NIPPV). A respiratory therapist comes out to Polly's apartment and fits a special mask over her nose. He then coaches her on how to accept the pressure of air from the ventilator, which is triggered when Polly takes a breath. Polly is grateful for this machine, since she is able to learn to sleep restfully at night.

Since no cause for the anemia/blood loss is known, and since Polly refuses further diagnostic workups, the case manager suggests that Polly's family donate blood, which can be transfused whenever Polly's hemoglobin drops below 10 grams. The case manager makes this suggestion to avoid future hospitalizations for the mysterious blood loss and to improve the quality of life for the patient.

Polly is grateful for the restful sleep and the strength she now has. She visits more frequently with her family. She feels she is going to die soon, although she does not discuss this with her children. One day she decides that it is time for her to go and that God should come and take her. She dies that very night.

CASE STUDY #5: SUBACUTE AND LONG-TERM CARE

George is a 66-year-old white man with no previous medical history. He smoked one to one and a half packs of cigarettes per day until two years ago, when he quit. He drinks one to two six-packs of beer on the weekends. He is 20 pounds overweight, and his liver enzymes are top normal. George presents to his primary care physician with the complaint of nocturia and urgency. A rectal exam reveals an enlarged prostrate and a urinary tract infection. The doctor refers George to a urologist, who explains the treatment options to George.

The urologist offers two options, watchful waiting or a transurethral resection of the prostrate (a TURP) to remove the bulk of the gland. He explains that there is little or no danger in waiting as long as George follows up on appointments. George elects to think about his decision. He later talks to his brother-in-law, who says that George's HMO wants to avoid surgery and that George should have the surgery because he paid his premiums and deserves it.

George elects to have surgery. He has a TURP, and requires continuous bladder irrigation postoperatively. The next morning George is restless and begins to complain of shortness of breath. He then has a melena stool, and within minutes is bleeding from every orifice. George evidently has disseminating intravascular coagulation (DIC), but before replacement blood can be prepared for transfusion, he goes into cardiac arrest.

George is resuscitated, but suffers from a stroke and apparent cerebral hypoxia as a result of the cardiac arrest. He is unable to articulate his needs and has some left-sided weakness. The HMO case manager finds a nursing home close to George's home that has opened a subacute care center. This center has selected stroke and elder dementia as part of its treatment offerings for patients who require intensive nursing care but do not require extensive diagnostic activity. The subacute care facility has a case manager who admits George to the facility, does an assessment of his needs, and interviews George's wife. A plan for rehabilitation and family teaching is put in place to prepare George for eventual discharge to home. At the end of a two-month stay, George is not cognizant of his surroundings and cannot care for himself. His wife decides that she cannot care for George at home and reluctantly seeks placement in the nursing home portion of the facility. George is later discharged from the subacute program and becomes a resident in the nursing home.

The case manager of the subacute facility is on hand to assess the appropriateness of the admission to the facility and to report progress to the HMO, the family, and the physician regarding George's care. When

George is ready for discharge to the nursing home portion, she makes the arrangements with the facility social worker and admissions clerk.

CASE STUDY #6: MANAGEMENT OF ASTHMA PATIENTS AS AN AT-RISK POPULATION

Asthma is a growing health problem in the United States, accounting for an estimated $6.2 billion in direct health expenditures and another $900 million in lost days at work and school.[1] Age-adjusted death rates grew 40 percent from 1980 to 1989, accounting for 4,867 deaths. Physician office visits for asthma grew from 6.5 million in 1985 to 7.1 million per year in 1990.[2]

Asthma seems to have multiple etiologic characteristics: familial, allergenic, socioeconomic, and environmental.[3] Lifestyle and psychological components also seem to be part of the equation, but there has been no adequate explanation for the rise in symptomatology or the fact that the rise in asthma is seen primarily among subgroups, mostly black males.

This case study involves a case management program for asthma patients. Part of the program is a built-in outcomes measurement process. There is a high cost to collecting outcomes data. This cost needs to be justified by the return on investment of case management dollars spent and reduction in the use of medical services and hospital visits. Identifying chronically ill patients and optimizing outcomes using health outcomes measures is also known as disease state management.

Linking Care across the Continuum: Home Care and Hospital

Home care agencies and hospitals are exploring ways to decrease the cost of care for their HMO customers and for their own strategic benefit. The following is an illustration of what a proprietary home care agency can do to provide services to a risk group of patients using case management. The collection of outcomes data is included in the service. Global goals for the risk population of asthma patients are

- reduced mortality
- reduced morbidity as measured by medical complications
- increased health-related behaviors as evidenced by decrease in cigarette smoking and more physically active lifestyle

- decreased respiratory symptoms: dyspnea, wheezing, cough, symptoms at night, symptoms during exercise
- improvement in physiologic airflow as measured by spirometry and peak flow
- increased functional capacity in terms of work/school attendance, ADLs
- improvement in self-rated quality of life: perception of well-being, physical functioning, mental and emotional functioning, social and role functioning
- decreased utilization of resources: ER visits, inpatient hospitalizations, physician office visits
- decreased other costs: drug costs, indirect costs of medical care, costs to family and employer

Since asthma is a chronic, lifelong condition that affects patients' quality of life if they are not actively involved in managing their own self-care, the strategy should include involving the patient and family to self-manage the condition as much as possible.

Steps of Collaborative Self-Care Management of Asthma

1. physical and functional assessment of patient status (physical exam, Health Status Questionnaire [HSQ], and Asthma TyPE specification from Health Outcomes Institute; see Chapter 6 for a further explanation of these tools)
2. development of treatment goals as shared by patient and clinician
3. discussion of the patient's concerns/fears/illness meanings
4. involvement of family as appropriate
5. development of a patient–clinician partnership that encourages communication and active patient participation; may include a contract
6. assessment of the patient's readiness to learn, including willingness and ability
7. instruction of the patient in a setting that maximizes comprehension and retention of material
8. assessment of the patient's knowledge and skill in self-care behaviors
9. repeated measures of HSQ/TyPE survey tool
10. planning of further interventions for outliers[4]

The strategic goals of the Hometime Healthcare Services agency are

- to become a major presence in home health services in the Philadelphia metropolitan region and southern New Jersey
- to prepare to satisfy managed-care organizations as major customers
- to collect outcomes data in the areas of
  1. cost—utilization of resources and capture of accurate billing data

2. access to care—response time and timeliness of service interventions
3. satisfation—patients, doctors, referral sources
4. health outcome—functional and clinical data that reflect service quality
5. productivity—of systems and people

The organizational goals of the company are

- to install outcomes measures to satisfy managed-care organization customers
- to become certified by Medicare and the Joint Commisssion for the Accreditation of Healthcare Organizations
- to demonstrate quality improvement (QI) processes that are congruent with Joint Commission Accreditation requirements
- to improve service capabilities
- to control cost variables
- to eliminate process deficiencies that lead to rework and lost productivity (billing on wrong form, miscoding, employee pay record errors, etc.)
- to capture nurses' notes from home health aides and eliminate lost revenues from visiting nurse associations
- to capture data that can be used to identify
  1. cost per patient
  2. cost per visit
  3. potential high-cost patients at beginning of health encounter
  4. functional and clinical outcomes of care
  5. patient/referral source/payer satisfaction
  6. satisfaction and health outcome per nurse
  7. all billable activity

The goals of the company include pleasing HMO customers, and to do that, the agency needs to implement an outcomes measurement effort. This effort has the additional effect of implementing a project that demonstrates to the Joint Commission that an active outcomes program is taking place, as mandated by their Performance Improvement standards. The goals of the agency's outcomes project are

1. to demonstrate commitment to managed-care organizations and the Joint Commission by starting a pilot project collecting outcomes measures with a select group of patients
2. to identify and train key personnel to carry out processes
3. to define data collection protocols, how information will be used and integrated into QI program, accounting and billing procedures

4. to integrate outcomes measures into QI program
5. to negotiate a risk/cost-sharing arrangement of outcomes measures start-up and data collection costs with managed-care organization customers
6. to set up policies, procedures, and equipment to collect outcomes measures
7. to perform a trial run to test and rework process

Exhibit 3–1 sets out some of the action steps that will require the use of consultant time. Exhibit 3–2 illustrates a budget for the project.

The costs of collecting the data for 300 patients per year, using in-person, mail, and phone encounters, are as follows:

First encounter: 30 minutes @ $50/hour = $25.00
Follow-up: mail (form + send and return postage) = $2.10
Follow-up phone (60% nonrespond, phone survey) 30 minutes @ $20/hr =
$10 x 60% = $6.00
Cost of initial, plus 3 follow-ups [$25 + (8.10 x 3)] = $49.30/patient
Overhead: Start-up cost and training, amortized over 3 years = $15,567/yr.
            Data manager and follow-up (0.4 FTE x $18,000)   7,200/yr.
            Equipment/software services   1,200/yr.

            Total $23,967/yr.
Overhead per patient (300 patients/year) $79.89 + $49.30 = $129.19/patient per year

The potential revenue and other costs to case-manage the asthma patients then are as follows:

Charge for service per patient: $ 390
Number of patients: 300
Revenue: $117,000
Costs: Outcomes data collection: 129.00
              Average 2 home visits   140.00
              Phone contact monthly   72.00
Total costs: $341.00
Net revenue: 49.00
Net profit ($49/$390): 12.5%

The data on emergency room visits, primary care, hospitalization costs, and so on are assumed to be collected by the HMO and provided to the home care agency as part of the effort to find out if the case management project is actually working.

Exhibit 3–3 shows return-on-investment (ROI) figures noted by the HMO for the asthma program. These figures are derived from a review of the asthma literature.[5] Note that the cost category that was least affected by case management was hospitalizations. It remains for the primary physician, the home care agency, and the hospital itself to tackle the problem by

Exhibit 3–1 Action Steps Required To Reach Project Goals

Task	Days Required
1. Brief key individuals: data manager, director of nursing	1
2. Work with QI personnel on outcomes measures and relation to Joint Commission and QI program	5
3. Support planning and negotiation with managed-care organizations regarding terms data collection	7
4. Plan interface of outcomes measures data with CFO	5
5. Plan and implement installation of system for data collection and storage	4
6. Train data manager and other responsible parties	4
7. Plan company-wide process for data collection, write policies/procedures	3
8. Do trial data collection and monitor	5
9. Set up data analysis with statistical consultant	2
10. Plan and implement full outcomes program for all patients	4
Total number of consulting days over four-month period	**40**

analyzing the data shown in Exhibit 3–3 and identifying a strategy to decrease the incidence and costs of hospitalizations. Their *next step* is to decrease incidence and cost of hospitalizations. The *critical clinical process* is airway and emotional management of the patient at the point of service. Their *strategy* is to institute a critical path in the emergency room in order to standardize the treatment of an acute asthmatic attack, to employ information systems support to identify patients with past history and find

Exhibit 3–2 Budget for Collection of Outcomes Data

	Price	Total/Category
Capital equipment		$6,900
486 PC with 250 MB HD & 12 MB RAM, color monitor	$3,900	
Scanner	$2,100	
Laser printer	$ 900	
Software		$5,000
Database software	$ 500	
Outcomes software and survey tools	$4,500	
Computer technical support		$2,800
Installation	$ 400	
Training of data manager and others	$1,200	
Health statistics programmer	$1,200	
Consulting administrator	40 days @$ 800	$32,000
Total		$46,700

out what interventions were used in the past with an individual patient, and to institute a critical path on-line that takes into account variances such as age and other comorbid factors.

Implementation of this strategy involves introducing new technology into the ER. One interesting and emerging technology for the treatment of acute respiratory distress is noninvasive positive pressure ventilation (NIPPV). This technology is made possible by small, easily maintained ventilators that are combined with tight-fitting nasal masks and the clinical expertise to fit the masks and coach the patient through the process of breathing through the mask instead of through his or her mouth. NIPPV is being used more in the home setting than the acute care setting, but numerous studies done in hospitals have noted its efficacy and safety.[6] Some of its advantages are decreased intubations, charges by anesthesiologists, pulmonary infections, days on ventilator, iatrogenic events (pneumothorax, tracheotomies, trauma to throat), and soft goods costs (suction catheters, etc.). Exhibit 3–4 lists indications for the use of NIPPV.[6]

Since anesthesia and respiratory departments in hospitals are still seen as revenue generators rather than cost centers, they depend on the more labor-intensive intubation and volume ventilator techniques of the past to manage the patient's airway. As hospital systems have changes forced upon them by the way they are reimbursed, the costs of doing things the old way will not be as acceptable.

NIPPV is a patient-focused intervention. This technology forces clinicians to design a treatment intervention based on the patient's own ability to move air. It is contingent on clinicians' ability to fit the mask, the airway

Exhibit 3–3 Return on Investment for Hometime Asthma Case Management

Type of Service	Cost Pre-CM	Cost Post-CM	% Change
Physician office visits (@$60/per)	72,000	36,000	–50
Medications (includes oral steroids			
and antibiotics)	142,000	56,800	–60
Emergency room visits (@$1500)	315,000	157,580	–50
Hospitalizations (@$5,400)	486,000	320,760	–34
Total	$1,015,000	571,140	
Cost of case management			
(300 x $390)	0	117,000	
Total costs with case management		688,060	–32
Savings		336,940	

Return on investment (ROI) for case management: $336,940/$117,000 = $2.88/$1.00

Exhibit 3–4 Indications for NIPPV

- **Acute Respiratory Insufficiency/Failure**
  1. respiratory acidosis
  2. respiratory distress
  3. use of accessory muscles or abdominal paradox
  4. patient cooperative
  5. patient hemodynamically stable
  6. intact airway, no excessive secretions
  7. proper mask fit achieved
- **Chronic Respiratory Insufficiency**
  1. obstructive sleep apnea
  2. upper airway resistance disease
  3. idiopathic hypoventilation
  4. neuromuscular disease
     (a) muscular dystrophies
     (b) postpolio syndrome
     (c) multiple sclerosis
     (d) amyotrophic lateral sclerosis
  5. thoracic wall deformities
     (a) kyphoscoliosis
     (b) post thoracoplasty

Note: Efficacy is not established in cases of chronic obstructive pulmonary disease. The intervention requires a cooperative and motivated patient who has minimal secretions.

pressures, the ventilator cycles, the patient's requirements, and an available 30 to 45 minutes to coach the patient through the acute process for the first time. Further, an alarm affixed to the ventilator will no longer work because the patient's own breathing cycle is too variable for most traditional alarm systems. The safety monitoring must be done by pulse oximetry, in which the patient rather than the machine is monitored, or by continual checking with the patient regarding his or her status.

BiPAP NIPPV uses a noncontinuous ventilator to augment patient ventilation. BiPAP is a biphisic mode of NIPPV. It involves a high inspiratory airway pressure and a lower pressure during the expiratory phase, both measured in centimeters of water. The cycle is based on patient effort, with a minimum of other settings. The patient has control over his or her own respiratory pattern. The inspiratory flow is regulated to match demand.

In our case study, a BiPAP NIPPV ventilation protocol is introduced into the ER. BiPAP in the ER is tolerated by 75% of patients at a cost of $2,000, and these patients are discharged within 24 hours. Lengths of stay for the remaining 15 patients decreases to five days at $1,000/day. As a result, costs decrease to $165,000/year for hospitalized patients.

In conclusion, asthma is a diagnostic category for which the care management is redesigned on the basis of case identification, case management, sorting out what the costs are, and bringing in new technology to make the care more efficient and effective. With this approach, the patients do better, the providers of home care and hospital care improve their efficiency and the patient outcome, and the payer works with providers who can lower the cost while improving the health outcome of the patient. The only losers are those who cannot adapt to the demands of the marketplace by making the care more efficient and effective.

NOTES

1. K. Weiss, An Economic Evaluation of Asthma in the United States, *New England Journal of Medicine* 326 (1992): 862.
2. Centers for Disease Control, Asthma—United States, 1980–1990, *Journal of the American Medical Association* 268 (1992):1995.
3. S. Wissow et al., Poverty, Race and Hospitalization for Childhood Asthma, *American Journal of Public Health* 78 (1988):777–82.
4. B. Make, Collaborative Self-Management Strategies for Patients with Respiratory Disease, *Respiratory Care* 39 (1994):567–583.
5. Make, Collaborative Self-Management Strategies.
6. T.J. Meyer and N.S. Hill, Noninvasive Positive Pressure Ventilation To Treat Respiratory Failure, *Annals of Internal Medicine* 120 (1994): 670–770.

4

Stretching Benefit Dollars: The Case Manager's Toolbox

COORDINATION OF BENEFITS

Due to multiple coverages and to block opportunity for fraud, there has been some effort to standardize coordination of benefits (COB) rules throughout the United States. A background knowledge of COB rules will assist case managers in various settings either to procure or to deny payment for services. Provider or advocacy case managers may find ways to stretch benefit dollars or recover payment for services already provided. Many insurance carriers treat coordination of benefits as a potential revenue source.

COB practice determines the way in which medical, dental, or other treatments should be paid when a patient is covered under more than one insurer. The National Association of Insurance Commissioners (NAIC) issued model regulations in 1970 with the goal of ensuring that payment for health services when more than one coverage was involved would not exceed 100 percent of the claim. Each state has its own COB rules, but many model their law after NAIC.[1]

Insurance carriers may choose to "pursue and pay" a claim—that is, check to see if there are any other coverages before paying a claim—or to "pay and pursue"—that is, attempt to collect on other coverages after the claim has already been paid. Health plans should have well-documented policies and procedures and consistent turnaround times for handling claims disputes.[2]

Allowable Expenses

Under NAIC guidelines, an *allowable expense* is any reasonable and customary (also called *U&C, usual and customary*) expense that is covered in whole or in part by any of the plans involved. An *eligible expense* is one that may be covered under one insurance contract but not another. Under COB rules, if the primary carrier permits payment for a service (considers it eligible), the secondary carrier must consider the expense allowable even though the expense was not eligible under their policy contract. Statements of medical necessity are important in COB determination of covered services.

Insurance Plans Included in COB

Insurance plans included in COB are

- group health insurance, including group type coverage through HMOs and other prepayment group practice plans
- automobile coverage for personal injury protection (PIP)
- Medicare and other government beneficiaries
- group or group-type hospital indemnity benefits that exceed $100 per day
- any group coverage and group subscriber contract

CHAMPUS and Medicaid plans are not included under COB rules. Plans created by the Employee Retirement Income Security Act of 1974 (ERISA plans) are permitted to have their own COB rules without interference from state law. There are special rules for coordination with HMOs and special cost containment contract provisions (e.g., benefit level reduced because precertification rules were not followed).

Benefits Bank

Secondary payers in COB can reduce their benefits so that these do not exceed 100 percent of the coverage. The excess is placed in a reserve category called a *benefits bank*. This money can be used to pay for allowable expenses that may not otherwise be covered.

Spousal and Dependent Coverage

According to NAIC rules, COB between divorced parents with dependent children pays out in the following sequence:

1. the plan of the parent in custody of the child
2. the plan of the spouse of the parent in custody of the child
3. the plan of the parent without custody of the children
4. the plan of the spouse without custody of the children

Special state rules apply when parents are divorced and separated so as to ensure coverage for the children.

Medicare Coverage

Medicare and Medicaid are the primary payers if it can be determined that the patient is eligible. They pay up to their fee schedule, and the secondary payer pays under the usual rules. Medicare is secondary payer to many employer-sponsored health plans, workers' compensation, and auto, liability, and no-fault coverage. Medicare is the primary payer of benefits when the individual becomes eligible for Medicare on the basis of his or her disability.

ERISA

The Employee Retirement Income Security Act of 1974 created a class of plans (ERISA plans) that were preempted from state (but not federal) laws governing insurance plans. There is no uniformity of COB among the ERISA plans, so employees and spouses are not given the protection of the state laws governing COB.

COBRA

The Consolidated Omnibus Budget Reconciliation Act of 1985 (P.L. 99-272), known as COBRA, provided legislation to ensure that employees who lost or changed their jobs could have continued health coverage for themselves, their spouses, and their dependents for a period of 18 months, provided they paid for the full cost of the coverage. Special qualifying events can extend this coverage up to 36 months. Many people keep COBRA coverage when they change jobs and have a pre-existing condition that requires a waiting period before new coverage comes into force.

ENTITLEMENTS AND ALTERNATIVE FUNDING SOURCES

Case managers should have a thorough understanding of the funding sources for the patients they are assisting, a general understanding of other sources, and a reference source for more detailed information as necessary. What follows is a general outline of some sources of funding that are entitled by federal law but that sometimes require an advocate who knows how to access the system in order to use the entitlement to gain coverage for the patient/client.

Medicare

Approximately 95 percent of the elderly are covered by Medicare insurance, which is funded by federal payroll taxes. Part A, mandatory hospital insurance (HI), pays for inpatient and posthospital skilled nursing services, home health care, and hospice care. Inpatient hospital care has a deductible, but the first 20 days of skilled care (i.e., nursing home or subacute care) do not. After that, the charge is $89.50 per day for days 21 through 100.

Medicare Part B, the supplementary medical insurance (SMI) program, is funded by voluntary participant premiums and general federal revenues. SMI covers physician services, outpatient hospital services, and some home health care. Medicare pays the provider 80 percent of the fee after a $100 deductible, which is based on the Resource Based Relative Value Schedule (RBRVS). The patient pays for the remaining 20 percent through Medigap insurance, out of pocket, or via Medicaid, if he or she is eligible. Medicare does not pay for prescriptions, dental care, eyeglasses, or long-term care.[3]

Medicaid

Medicaid is funded jointly by federal, state, and local governments. The federal government sets the minimum eligibility requirements, and each state designs the scope of the services to meet its own needs and budget. About one-third of the national Medicaid budget was spent on long-term care nationally, and almost 40 percent went to hospital care for the poor. Medicaid is the largest third-party payer for long-term care, making up 45 percent of its revenues in 1990.[4]

Medicaid coverage does not guarantee access to care. One study found that 20 percent of adults have trouble getting and paying for care. Many Medicaid beneficiaries have trouble accessing the basic necessities of life.[5] State governments are looking to Medicaid managed-care organizations to limit the enormous cost of this entitled program. But whereas for-profit HMOs have hospitalization rates per 1,000 covered lives down to about 150 days (range 120–180) per year (e.g., 30 hospitalizations with a length of stay of 5 days = 150), Medicaid HMOs have annual hospitalization usage for 1,000 people at about 1,200 days per year. Approximately 90 percent of the admissions are via hospital emergency rooms.

Currently, about 200 HMOs provide health coverage to some four million Medicaid enrollees. It is expected that by 1996, most states will have managed Medicaid.[6]

Medicaid Waiver Programs

Medicaid waiver programs are an important alternative funding source for case managers to be aware of. The details of most of these waiver programs are known to social workers who are employed by the state. Medicaid waiver programs were set up to fulfill the Omnibus Budget Reconciliation Act of 1981, Section 2176, Public Law 97-35, and amendments under Public Law 99-509, which encouraged the development of community-based services for those who were in need of long-term institutional care. The purpose of the legislation is to enable eligible individuals to remain in or return to a community setting instead of being cared for in an institution. The name of these programs comes from the fact that the federal requirement for institutional care is "waived" for the special circumstances.

Waiver programs must be cost-neutral or cost-effective, meaning that the state has to pay amounts to providers for the care of the eligible individuals that are equal to or less than the costs of long-term institutional care. Individuals eligible for SSI or SSDI and within certain age, asset, and income categories are eligible for the programs. The state contracts with private providers to render the care in most cases.

There are two types of waiver programs, regular and model waivers. Regular waivers are aimed at risk populations aged 65 and older, those with developmental or acquired disabilities and chronic illnesses who require more than 2.5 hours of nursing care a day. These individuals are entitled to case management, homemaker services, transportation services, special medications, medical day care, and a number of other services. The range of services is specified in the provisions of each program. Model waiver programs include special diagnoses, such as AIDS, TBI, or blindness.[7]

Each state shares responsibility with the federal government on a 50-50 basis for the funding of the programs as approved by the Health Care Financing Administration. Funding for each program lasts from three to five years. The state considers itself the payer of last resort. A limited number of slots are funded in each state. Finding out about the specifics of each state's waiver program can be difficult. The National Association for Home Care produces a list of Medicaid waiver programs for each state.[8] Each state's health and social service department has overall responsibility for Medicaid waiver programs.

Case managers (usually social workers) have the responsibility of writing the plan of care and 24-hour coordination of the plan of care. They assist in deciding who is eligible and what services individuals should receive according to the specifications of the program. They are responsible for ensuring the quality of the service delivered by the provider organizations.

Entitlements by Civil Rights Statutes

A progressive series of legislation and legal precedent (case law) has affirmed constitutionally guaranteed civil rights. The Civil Rights Act of 1964 specifically prohibits discrimination in places of "public accommodation." The constitutional basis for this act is the power of Congress to regulate interstate commerce, and due to Supreme Court decisions that date back to the 1930s, nearly all economic activity can be legally classified as interstate commerce.[9] Thus, any activity between people in a public setting can be considered commerce, and certain standards of behaviors can be set.

Americans with Disabilities Act

The Americans with Disabilities Act of 1990 (ADA; P.L. 101-336), signed into law by President Bush, was designed to provide access to public accommodation so that the federal government could limit the enormous ($150 billion yearly) cost of long-term disability paid out by the Social

Security Administration. Present disabled children are future disabled adults.

Attorney General Dick Thornburgh wrote in an introduction to a U.S. government pamphlet explaining the ADA:

> Barriers to employment, transportation, public accommodations, public services and telecommunications have imposed staggering economic and social costs on American society and have undermined our well-intentioned efforts to educate, rehabilitate, and employ individuals with disabilities.[10]

Both Republicans and Democrats moved to mandate fundamentally increased rights of Americans to have access to services that would empower them because it was much cheaper for society to do so.

Definition of Disability. A *disability* is a physical or mental impairment that substantially limits a major life activity. *Substantially limits* means that the individual cannot perform a major life activity under the conditions, in the manner, or for the duration that a normal person could perform the given activity. *Major life activity* is also measured by what a normal person would do in terms of activities of daily living and broad categories of occupation.

Scope of the Legislation. Title I regulates access to employment. Discrimination is prohibited in the full range of employment activities, including job application procedures, hiring and discharge procedures, level of compensation, job training, and advancement.

A prospective employee can be tested for competitive employment only regarding actual or essential functions of the job. If the employment candidate has problems with access to the facility or its amenities (bathrooms, doors, etc.), this should not be a barrier to employment. The employer must make his or her facility and performance of the job accessible to a reasonable degree.

Employers who have changed their job descriptions to be in compliance with Title I have reviewed the job objectives and functions, including quantifying work tasks in a way that identifies risks of injury to those who may be at risk for disability (e.g., warehouse workers with a previous history of a back injury cannot be denied employment but must be given reasonable accommodation, or protection, from reinjury).

All employers with at least 15 employees are now subject to the provisions of Title I.

Title II covers access to all public services, including transportation. It regulates all public transportation and was written to phase in more responsive paratransit systems.

Title III focuses on access to public accommodations. This is the most visible section of the law in terms of ramp access to buildings, automatic doors, and other changes in access so that any business or place that is otherwise open to the public accommodates all.

Interestingly, Title III of the ADA actually uses the term *commerce* rather than *public accommodation* in order to broaden the rules of application. Sections 302(a) and 302(b)(1) address discriminatory denials of access or participation and the provision of unequal benefits, and encourage the participation of individuals with disabilities in the most integrated setting appropriate to their needs. Section 36.201(a) contains the general rule that prohibits discrimination on the basis of disability in the full and equal enjoyment of goods, services, facilities, privileges, advantages, and accommodations of any place of public accommodation (28 CFR Part 36, Dept. of Justice; *Federal Register*, Vol. 56, No. 144, July 26, 1991).

According to Section 36.212, insurance companies may offer insurance policies that limit coverage for certain procedures or treatments, but may not deny coverage to a person with a disability. Also,

> The plan may not refuse to insure, or limit the amount, extent, or kind of coverage available to an individual, or charge a different rate for the same coverage solely because of a physical or mental impairment, except where the refusal, limitation or rate differential is based on sound actuarial principles.

Section 36.212 was adopted into the rulemaking without change, due to the variability of comments to federal rulemakers. Section 36.302 takes the logic one step further by ruling that "a public accommodation shall make reasonable modifications in policies, practices or procedures, when the modifications are necessary to afford goods, services, facilities, privileges, advantages, or accommodations to individuals with disabilities."

Court cases to test the law and Justice Department action against municipalities who have not yet complied with the law are in the beginning phases. (It seems that it is not easy to get many disabled people to go through the court procedures to challenge this issue.)

One issue in the future may be payment for health interventions that are not deemed necessary by utilization reviewers because the person has a chronic disease or disability. Denial of payment for Medicare home health services on the grounds that they constitute chronic care may be similarly challenged.

Title IV was designed to bring telephone services to the 24 million hearing-impaired and 2.8 million speech-impaired people in the United

States. Continuous operation of 24-hour-a-day telecommunication relay service throughout the United States is the eventual goal.

Title V contains miscellaneous provisions, including stipulations on insurance coverage and underwriting practice. It authorizes reasonable fees to be paid to attorneys, including litigation expenses and costs to the prevailing party. Although drug and alcohol use are considered disabilities under the ADA, the ADA does not protect anyone involved in illegal drug use from being discharged. Other exclusions and disorders not protected under ADA statute are sexual behavioral disorders, gambling, and kleptomania. Homosexuality and bisexuality are specifically not considered impairments or disabilities.

Individuals with Disabilities Education Act

The Individuals with Disabilities Education Act of 1991 (IDEA; P.L. 101-476), extended the provisions of the All Handicapped Children Act of 1975, which required states receiving federal monies for public education to provide free appropriate public education and related services to children with developmental disabilities from birth to age 21 or the completion of high school.

The right of due process for parents is built into the law. Each state must have procedures to appeal the decisions of the local school superintendent. This right is backed up by the right of the parents to sue in federal court, with the school district compelled to reimburse parents' attorney fees and pay expert witness costs if they lose. The procedures for enrolling and testing in each state differ, but the basic principles provide a structure for due process for the parents to ensure that their child can get the services needed to attempt to minimize his or her impairment or disability.

Eligibility Requirements. All children who are physically and/or mentally impaired and require special attention in order to learn are eligible to receive special educational benefits.

Children from birth to age three are eligible for early intervention services if they have a developmental delay or a physical or mental disability that is likely to result in developmental delay. The term *developmental delay* includes such areas as physical, language and speech, cognitive, emotional, and social development. Depending on the regulations in each state, the services may have to be delivered by the local social services system, or the parents may be able to request an individualized program that is cheaper for the state and more beneficial for the child.

Early intervention services usually include such categories as physical and speech therapy, psychological services, and specialized learning instruction. Assistance is provided on a case-by-case basis, so the parents must state their case for the program that they wish to utilize.

Children from ages three to five are evaluated at least yearly to determine their level of physical and developmental disability. The local school district should have an expert team of educators and psychologists in place to aid with the evaluations. The parents need a local expert (their doctor, an educational or developmental disabilities expert, etc.) to assist in their dealings with the school district.

For *children from ages 5 to 21*, the school district must prepare and adhere to an individualized educational plan (IEP). The child must first be identified as "exceptional" by the school district. To be judged exceptional, the child must have at least one of the following physical, mental, or emotional conditions and have documentation of these conditions by qualified health professionals using the appropriate objective tests:

- *Brain damage or injury*: Defined as a severe insult to the brain that is identified by a neurological evaluation and that causes severe behavior and learning disorders. The mechanism or cause of the injury is not relevant to qualify for benefits. What is important is the documentation of the injury and the resultant disability.
- *Mental retardation*: Impaired mental functioning, with an IQ of below 80 or a problem learning in a standard educational setting.
- *Physical handicaps*: Impairments that limit a child's accommodation to a classroom setting and interfere with educational performance. Severely handicapped children are defined as having two or more of the following conditions: blindness, brain damage, cerebral palsy, deafness, emotional disturbance, muscular dystrophy, and severe mental retardation.
- *Social and emotional disturbances*: Display of unacceptable behavioral characteristics over an extended period of time. This category can include those children with attention deficit disorder.
- *Speech and language impairments*: Disorders that impair academic achievement and are due to language, voice, and speech articulation.

The Individualized Educational Plan. The IEP is a document resulting from a process that begins when the parents apply to the school district to have special attention given to their child's needs (see Appendix 4–A for a sample letter). The documentation of the child's doctor is submitted, along with the suggested course of action (treatment plan) that will address the child's problems. The school district will have their own expert examine the child to document the extent of the alleged disability. They generally have someone on their staff or someone who does these evaluations for them. The specialist who examines the child should have the appropriate level of expertise related to the child's disability.

After the initial evaluation by the school district's expert, a multidisciplinary team of educators in the school district makes a judgment on the "exceptionality" of the child, then generally construct an IEP based on their evaluation of the child's needs. The IEP must include

1. a statement of the child's present level of educational performance
2. a statement of annual goals that describes the expected behaviors to be achieved through the child's IEP
3. a statement of short-term instructional objectives
4. a statement of specific educational services to be provided to the child, including a description of all special educational and related services required to meet the unique needs of the child, any special instructional material required, and the type of physical education program in which the child will participate
5. a description of the extent to which the child will be able to participate in regular educational programs
6. the projected date of initiation and expected duration of the services
7. a statement of the evaluation procedures and schedules for determining whether the educational objectives are being realized (assessments must be made at least annually)

The multidisciplinary team, the parents, and any expert (and attorney) that is brought to the process by the parents meet to agree on the IEP. The document generated is a legally enforceable contract in that the school district must provide (or cause to be provided) the services that are set forth in it.

Often the negotiations over what the school district will provide bog down over the issue of "related services." The services generally covered under related services include transportation to and from school, specialized equipment such as wheelchairs or ramps, speech pathology, audiology, psychological services, physical therapy, occupational therapy, and other services related to the child's developmental issues.[11]

The class structure recommended in the IEP can range from home instruction assisted by a teacher who comes to the house for five or more hours per week, to special education classes, to "mainstreaming" of the child in regular classroom settings. The case law precedents under this statute tend to support parents who wish to mainstream their child. The parents should attempt to arrange for services that will enable the child to obtain his or her highest level of physical, mental, and emotional functioning. The aim of the educational focus and the therapy is to mainstream the child at the least resource cost to the school district. It is not unusual for the school district to place the child in a private, special school when they do not have the resources to fund a full program for all their special education students.

Making the Process Work for the Child. To make this process work, one must understand the motivations of the participants. *School district* personnel are charged with providing for their students within a budget, and the biggest issue for them in coming to grips with an IEP is the cost in terms of their time and the money spent by the district. The family needs to clarify the official written policy with the school district and in some cases with the state in order to get a reasonable picture of how the system works. Parents need to watch out for hidden agendas among school district officials.

The *educational experts* used by the school district have a bias based on their training and their view of their role in the process. They may need to justify their existence as gatekeepers to the process. The parents should find out the school district educators' philosophy and opinions concerning their role in developing the IEP.

The *parents of the child* wish to obtain the best educational and functional outcome for their child, while minimizing their out-of-pocket expenses. They must convince school officials that their chosen course of action is best for the child *and* the school district. Additionally, this course of action must fulfill the letter and spirit of the law and limit the federal government's exposure to long-term disability costs under the Social Security Act.

Given the motivations of the above participants, individual strategies can be devised to gain access to a reasonable level of funding for a child's life of education. A collaborative process in devising an appropriate IEP can enhance the child's chance of going forward with a program that is beneficial for the child rather than easy to administer by the school district. The expected outcome and expenses of the school district's plan and the parents' plan can be compared for cost and quality. *Quality* is defined as a quantitatively higher level of physical, developmental, and educational functioning by the child.

If for any reason school district officials do not negotiate their position in good faith or obstruct the process, it may be wise to engage an attorney who has expertise in the local interpretation of the IDEA statute.

A reasonable budget should be drawn up, including the costs of visits, telephone consultations, home schooling, and any support services that are foreseen as necessary to optimize the outcome.

Timelines for Developing and Implementing an IEP. Within three months of the date of the parents' request or consent, a child should be referred to the child study team and evaluated, and a preliminary plan should be developed and implemented. The basic portion of the IEP should be drawn up within a month of the date that the child was declared disabled and the school district acknowledged responsibility. The basic plan should be implemented within a month of the plan's acceptance by all parties.

If there is a dispute concerning the plan that cannot be resolved, a mediator can be requested. In some cases, an administrative law judge may be required to hold a hearing. A judgment should be forthcoming from the mediator or judge within a reasonable (30-day) period. Due process procedures are as follows:

1. *Prehearing conference*: Parents request in writing an informal conference to attempt to resolve or settle a disagreement. (See Appendix 4–A for a sample letter).
2. *Due process hearing*: Takes place before a mediator or hearing officer assigned by the state. The parents may be represented by a lawyer or other person. Evidence can be presented so as to document the parents' position concerning the specialized needs of the child that the school district is not willing or able to meet. (See Appendix 4–A for a sample letter requesting a hearing.)
3. *Appeal*: Due process dictates that parents can appeal the decision of the hearing officer in state or federal court.

Other Sources for Funding Health Care

Many associations, voluntary organizations, and self-help societies throughout the United States provide information on a variety of illness conditions, from alopecia to vertigo. The best place to find these sources is the *Case Management Resource Guide*.[12] Professional and trade organizations, computer databases, state agencies, and programs are also listed. National self-help societies have many local chapters that one can access by calling the national society. Another good source of information is the National Association for Rare Diseases and Orphan Drugs in Washington, D.C., (800) 456-3505.

USE OF ALTERNATIVE MEDICINE

Alternative medicine comprises nonallopathic interventions that are noninvasive, may arise from cultural or religious traditions, and are generally not reimbursable by third-party payers. Such treatments as naturopathy, various massage techniques, chiropractic, acupuncture, midwifery, celation, diets, herbs, and the laying on of hands come under the heading of alternative therapies. Because there is no social sanction given by third-party payers and no listing in the physician-controlled CPT (Current Procedural Terminology) Book, these therapies are generally paid for out of pocket. In some cases, it may be beneficial to the payer and the patient to follow an alternative treatment when there is no viable alternative and the patient/family requests the therapy. In this case, an out-of-contract agreement will have to be initiated unless the insurance plan already has provisions for the payment of such therapies.

Some regional insurers and HMOs allow for traditional healers or payment for herbal remedies because they cost so much less and provide symptomatic relief in cases for which allopathic medicine has no answers.[13] Alternative treatments are generally nontoxic or do not interfere with allopathic treatments. For this reason they are sometimes called *complementary* treatments. Use of these interventions should be guided by the following conditions:

1. They are initiated by the patient/family.
2. There are few viable choices of other therapy, or the therapy is part of a cultural tradition.
3. The alternative/complementary treatment will not interfere with the ongoing course of treatment or otherwise harm the patient.
4. Outcome expectations are clearly stated, and intensiveness of treatment is clearly prescribed and preapproved.

OUT-OF-CONTRACT AGREEMENTS

Generally, out-of-contract arrangements are made to bring resources to bear when the policy does not cover the proposed therapy or equipment but the patient would clearly benefit from the proposed intervention. Insurance companies will generally agree to out-of-contract interventions when they are cost-neutral or cost-effective (i.e., they would cost less).

The case manager must formally propose the course of action and project cost savings to the payer in order to open negotiations for such a settlement. A statement that the out-of-contract service is not usually covered in the provisions of the policy, the reasons for the change, and the expected benefit to the patient should be set down as part of the out-of-contract agreement.

VIATICAL SETTLEMENTS

Viatical settlements are contracts to sell the value of a person's life insurance so as to gain access to money to pay for services for a terminally ill patient. The viatical company essentially buys the face value of the person's life insurance policy. The terms of the settlement include

- diagnosis of a terminal illness
- case reviewed by viatical settlement company doctors
- valuation of policy dependent on present interest rates, the premium obligation currently existing, and the life expectancy of the individual

Viatical settlement companies are generally divisions of insurance companies. The valuation of the policy is negotiated so that there is value in researching different companies and bargaining over the actual amount to be paid for the policy.

CASE STUDY #1: ARCHITECTURAL ADAPTATIONS

Under some circumstances, a case manager will be called on to be involved in adapting a home environment for a severely injured and disabled individual. A number of issues are pertinent here: access and egress to the dwelling, unimpeded movement throughout the living quarters, and safety, especially in the bathroom and in tub and toilet transfers. Many rehabilitation facilities have staff who have training and experience doing architectural assessments, and some construction firms now specialize in this area, especially since the passage of the ADA legislation.

The following case study was done at the request of the PIP carrier. The parents of the injured person requested an addition to their house so as to improve the access and quality of life of their son. The home had been modified previously, with the insurance carrier paying for the improvements, but some of the situations were not adequately addressed because the contractor had no experience with planning for a wheelchair-disabled individual.

This case involves a 28-year-old male injured in a pickup truck accident at age 19, nine years prior. His chronic neurogenic pain and spasm were felt by the family to be made worse by noise and his bedroom environment, which could not be finely controlled.

The family doctor wrote to the insurance company on behalf of the parents with the following issues:

- Noise from the next-door trucking company was disturbing the claimant's sleep early in the morning and leading to increased pain and neurogenic spasm.
- The claimant's room was too warm in summer and too cold in winter, causing spasm. The window air conditioner was not a good solution

because the claimant could not control it automatically, because it tended to block what little vision he had of the outside world, and because the cool air would blow directly on him.

- There was not enough room for storage of equipment in the present room.
- The claimant had no privacy when he had to be toileted since he had to leave his room and go into the bathroom, and these rooms were next to the living room.
- The aging parents did not feel capable of safely transferring their son from the bed to the wheelchair.

The claimant was seen at his residence, and the parents were interviewed. The findings are contained in the rehabilitation initial evaluation report (Appendix 4–B). The doctor was also interviewed by phone. He estimated the life span of the patient to be approximately ten more years, due to the inability of the claimant to take in adequate food, secondary to his chronic neurogenic dysreflexia pain.

The room was examined, and measurements of the room and adjacent bathroom were obtained (see Exhibits A and B in Appendix 4–B). The room was set up so that the claimant could see his dressers, which contained many personal items set up by his mother, such as family pictures. The setup appeared cluttered.

A building contractor was engaged to examine the room and bathroom. The drawing in Exhibit B was given to the contractor with the charge that the rooms be soundproofed and adapted for better environmental (heating and cooling) control. The resulting solution is shown in the evaluation report. The estimate of the cost of the renovations over the expected life of the patient came to under $800 per year. This compromise enabled the claimant, family, and the insurance company to feel that a win-win solution had been obtained.

CASE STUDY #2: A LIFE CARE PLAN

Life care plans are drawn up for the purpose of predicting the costs of care over a person's lifetime. They are done for the purpose of negotiating settlements and as a basis for asking for damages where injury has occurred. Rehabilitation case managers sometimes specialize in life care plans and may be required to appear in court to defend or explain a plan and its cost categories.

The case study here, a composite of several actual cases, presents many of the issues that arise in catastrophic spinal cord injury (SCI). The story is that of a young man who was injured by an automobile at age 13 and suffered an incomplete SCI to C4/C5. Martin Trent was hospitalized and had an anterior cervical fusion done with halo traction, went through a long course of physical therapy, and eventually went home to a motorized wheelchair that he maneuvered using a joystick with his left hand. He was able to stand and pivot with maximal assist and required three hours of nursing care a day plus his parents' help. He also required a skilled visit in the evening to catheterize him when the family was unavailable.

Martin adjusted to his injury and had a high quality of life by his own standards. He completed high school and college. He had a job at home utilizing his computer and had a girlfriend. He was able to travel independently in his van and had friends from all over the East Coast who traveled in a similar fashion.

At age 25, Martin was involved in a motor vehicle accident in which he was hit on the side of the vehicle, sustaining a small laceration on his head and some complaint of abdominal pain secondary to the lapbelt portion of the seat belt. Martin was boarded using a hard collar from the accident as per protocol, and C-spine films were negative in the emergency room (done as a precaution with the given history). However, over the next 60 days, Martin gradually lost the use of his left hand. The MRI showed no findings different from a preaccident film, but the second accident had completed the injury so that Martin was not able to do the most basic things for himself. Compounding this issue, his parents were no longer able to care for him due to their age and health status. Martin now needed 24-hour-a-day care, as he was unable even to shift his position in bed.

In preparing the file for court, an investigation was done to determine past and future costs of care and to estimate the fault involved from the first to the second accident so as to apportion responsibility and settlement between insurance companies.

Medical records from all the treating providers were reviewed. An additional medical exam was performed to establish the extent of the injury. A neurologist who saw Martin after the first accident was asked to re-evaluate the patient now that the second accident had significantly changed his status, compare his records to the preinjury exam, and make certain judgments about his injury, his functional capacity, his longevity, and his quality of life. Exhibit 4–1 shows the letter to the neurologist.

The rehabilitation consultant's report (Appendix 4–C) provides a commentary on the life care plan. The life care plan (Appendix 4–D) was based on some of the information provided by the neurologist, as well as a record

Exhibit 4–1 Case Study #2: Letter Requesting Neurologist's Re-Evaluation

November 20, 1994

Stanley Tourper, M.D.
Old South Rehabilitation Hospital
Columbia, SC
RE: Martin Trent
DOL: 11/16/81 & 12/14/93

Dear Dr. Tourper:

I am a rehabilitation nurse who has been asked by the above-captioned patient and his attorney to assist them with determining medical issues resulting from the above-captioned losses from motor vehicle accidents. Since you last saw Mr. Trent in 1987, he sustained injuries that further decreased his ability to function and his quality of life.

Mr. Trent will be calling you for an appointment for an examination. In this exam, I would ask you to determine the following:

1. Please determine how his present physical and functional condition compares and differs from his exam in 1987.
2. Please estimate his life span and treatment needs so that a life care plan can be constructed. Please estimate his life span and functional abilities had he *not* suffered the second accident of 12/14/93.
3. Please attribute the extent of the injuries between the first accident and the second one.
4. Please give an opinion as to any surgical or medical interventions that would improve his condition or quality of life.
5. Mr. Trent was working prior to the accident of 12/14/94. Please give an opinion as to his capacity to work after the accident.

I would like to attend this examination so that we can be assured that all pertinent issues are covered. I look forward to meeting with you.

Sincerely,

Michael Newell, RN, MSN, CCM

cc: Martin Trent
plaintiff attorney

of previous expenses related to the care of this individual. The figures in the life plan were later projected over the lifetime of the claimant so as to arrive at a figure for the monetary exposure of the insurance companies for the care of this claimant. An economist was contracted to project the future value of the listed services.

NOTES

1. T. Holloway et al., *The Coordination of Benefits Handbook* (Washington, D.C.: Thompson Publishing Group, 1995).
2. E.B. Pascuzzi, Claims and Benefits Administration, in *The Managed Health Care Handbook*, 2nd ed., ed. P. Kongstvedt (Gaithersburg, Md.: Aspen Publishers, Inc., 1993), 227–228.
3. C. Polich et al., *Managing Health Care for the Elderly* (New York: John Wiley & Sons, Inc., 1993), 25–27.
4. Polich, *Managing Health Care for the Elderly*, 28.
5. J. Blendon et al., DATAWATCH: Medicaid Beneficiaries and Health Reform, *Health Affairs* 12 (1993):132–143.
6. J. Coleman, MCO Trends, *The Case Manager* 4, no. 4 (1993):36–37.
7. D. Hartz, A Brief Overview of Home and Community Based Service Programs (Paper presented at the conference "Chronic Disease Management," East Brunswick, N.J., June, 1994).
8. National Association for Home Care, *Medicaid Waivers State-By-State*, 2nd ed.(Washington, D.C.:1993).
9. A.F. Southwick, *The Law of Hospital and Healthcare Administration*, 2nd. ed. (Ann Arbor, Mich.: Health Administration Press, 1988), 301–304.
10. *The Americans with Disabilities Act: Questions and Answers* (Washington, D.C.: Government Printing Office, 1991).
11. J.L. Romano, *Legal Rights of the Catastrophically Ill and Injured: Planning for the Future*, 4th ed. (Conshohocken, Pa.: Rosenstein & Romano, 1993), 45–56.
12. Center for Consumer Healthcare Information, *Case Management Resource Guide* (Irvine, Calif.: 1994). Published yearly, with regional volumes. Lists providers of care, equipment and other resources that may be used by case managers. Phone orders: (800) 627-2244.
13. B. Carton, Health Insurers Embrace Eye-of-Newt Therapy, *Wall Street Journal*, January 30, 1995, B1.

Appendix 4–A

Sample Letters from Parents Regarding Special-Needs Education

❧❦❧

REQUEST FOR EVALUATION

Principal's Name
School Name
School Address

Dear_____:

I am the parent of_____, age_____, who is a student in grade_____at
_____School. I have reason to believe that my child has special needs that cannot be met by the regular school program. [Explain briefly why you believe this to be true.] Please arrange to have my child evaluated by a child study team so that an appropriate program can be provided. Thank you.

Sincerely yours,
(parent's name)

REQUEST FOR MEDIATION

Division of Special Education
Department of Education
Anystate, USA

Dear:

I am the parent of_____, age_____, who is currently a student at the _____School in the _____District of Anystate. I have met with the representatives of the school district, but we have been unable to resolve a disagreement regarding my son/daughter's education. The disagreement involves [explain *briefly* the issue to be discussed at the mediation]. I am therefore requesting that a mediation conference be scheduled where we can discuss this matter and attempt to resolve it.

Sincerely yours,
(parent's name)

cc: Superintendent of Schools

REQUEST FOR A HEARING

Division of Special Education
Department of Education
Anystate, USA

Dear_____:

I am the parent of_____, age_____, who is a student at the
_____School in the District of Anystate. I have met with represen-
tatives of the school district, but we have been unable to resolve a disagreement regarding the proposed program. The disagreement involves [ex-
plain *briefly* the issue to be discussed at the hearing]. I am therefore
requesting that a due process hearing be scheduled so that the matter can
be resolved. Thank you.

Sincerely yours,
(parent's name)

cc: Superintendent of Schools

Appendix 4–B

Case Study #1: Rehabilitation
Initial Evaluation Report

To: Steven Adjuster
From: Michael Newell, RN, MSN, CCM
Report Date: 5/18/94

File: A3327-06721
Claimant: Thomas Logan
DOL: 12/6/85

Initial Evaluation

Mr. Thomas Logan was referred for evaluation because of a request by the family and physician to improve the living conditions of the claimant secondary to injuries that left him severely disabled. The available medical record was reviewed, and the patient and parents were interviewed at their home in order to evaluate the needs and estimate the costs of performing modifications to the home that would fairly address the requests of the family and physician.

Profile

Name: Thomas Logan
Address: 196 Pennsylvania Ave
         Johnstown, PA
Height/weight: 5'10", 110 lbs.

Age: 28
Telephone: 825-0321

DOB: 3/11/66

Brief History of Events

Mr. Logan was found unconscious at the scene of a motor vehicle accident on 12/6/85. Patient was areflexic of extremities and was found to have a C5 cord injury. Patient required a halo traction to stabilize spinal cord. He also had an evacuation of a subdural hematoma. He was discharged to Placebo Rehabilitation Institute on 2/23/86 with severe bedsores that required skin flaps to close. The patient was discharged to home on 7/19/86. The family and patient state that there was very little rehabilitation done and that his pain during that time hampered such efforts.

The patient later had a dorsal column implant done at the Hospital of Universal Prestige in September 1986, but it never worked properly. Subsequently, he had a mylogram at HUP that caused his sensation of spinal pain and spasm of the trunk to be appreciably worse, such that he still describes his pain to be 10/10 most of the time and to be worse when he talks, eats anything more than a little bit, or is disturbed by environmental stressors such as cold, heat, or noise. In 1988 he had a dorsal reentry zoning procedure done at University Hospital for the relief of pain. This procedure was unsuccessful in achieving this goal.

The patient has had several hospitalizations since for kidney lithotripsy and for urinary tract infections and has been followed by a urologist. The urologist changes the foley catheter every six weeks because of the bladder stricture. The patient is currently on antibiotics for bladder infection, which he and the family describe as constant. He states that he is trying to stay out of hospitals because he "was almost killed" on several occasions. He is seen approximately every four months in his home by Dr. Jones for his general medical care. The patient is currently on IM Gentamycin for his urinary tract infection and Valium 5 mg PO at night for spinal cord spasm and pain, but the patient states that the valium brings him no relief.

Mr. Logan has limited use of both arms. He can position his hands and push buttons. He currently possesses a device that can work the controls for lights, television, and a small portable heater in his bedroom. He keeps his legs flexed so as to reduce the spasm, but this limits the flexibility of his legs further. He spends all of his time in bed except for his morning bath. He leaves the house only to visit doctors, as it is extremely painful for him to be transported. He does not use a wheelchair at home except to transport outside to the car. He does not appear to be a candidate for any rehabilitation and could not tolerate any such effort due to the pain.

Current Problems

1. spinal cord injury at C5 with quadriplegia
2. S/P evacuation of right subdural hematoma
3. neurogenic bowel and bladder
4. chronic urinary tract infections
5. chronic pain syndrome
6. cachexia

On April 20, 1994, Dr. Jones wrote a letter to the insurance company listing some issues regarding the patient's room set-up. He listed lack of storage space, difficult access to the room due to 30-inch doorway, lack of privacy to the bathroom, and lack of discrete temperature control, which affects his spinal cord spasm and thus his pain sensation. Our visit with the patient and family also covered these issues and the issue of a trucking business next door to the Logan residence that causes extremely loud noises, often in the early morning and at unpredictable times. The family requests moving the patient's bedroom to the other side of the house or otherwise soundproofing the patient's room.

Provider Contact

Dr. Jones was subsequently interviewed by telephone. He has known the patient for 18 months. He estimates the patient's expected life, given the circumstances, to be another ten years. He reiterated the issues outlined in his letter during the conservation.

The requests made for the patient by the doctor and his family are as follows:

1. a Hoyer lift to transport the patient out of bed
2. more room so that the patient has storage available to him
3. access to the bathroom that gives the patient privacy
4. better temperature control in the room
5. an absence of noise from the next-door neighbors, who cause trucks and other equipment to be used at inconvenient times of the day and night

There was the general expectation that these issues could only be addressed by construction of a new room on the other side of the house. Dr. Jones stated in his letter that the patient is unable to gain access in and out of the house by himself. However, the patient has not been able to be self-mobile in the past, and there is no hope that he will be able to be in the future.

Proposed Solution

All of the issues raised by the family and the doctor, with the exception of the patient's mobility, can be addressed by modification in the existing rooms without the need for new construction. The issues, solutions, and cost estimates are found in Table A. Exhibits A and B illustrate the room layouts. The figures in Table A were obtained from two builders, including O.K. Construction, who surveyed the situation some months ago at the behest of the insurance carrier. Note that the soundproofing issues may not be the responsibility of the insurance company to handle, since the condition of the noise next door is not directly attributable to the accident. The family might install signs in English and Spanish regarding behaviors, or seek civil remedies.

Total cost of suggested remedies per year of life expectancy: $7,950.

Table A Room Modification Estimates

Issue	Solution	Cost Estimate
Bathroom door/privacy	Move bathroom door/close hallway door, relocate plumbing in BR to accomplish this	$1,850
Lack of space in room/ storage	Reconfigure bed/furniture setup in room (see Exhibits A and B)	no cost
Inadequate temperature control in room/unable to be controlled by patient	Install "split-type" AC/heat pump with remote control	$3,750 (includes new 220 electric line)
Noise from next door	Remove window on south side of house, install larger double- or triple-glazed window on east side of house, install drywall on 2 walls to soundproof	$1,500
Hoyer lift	Purchase	$850
	TOTAL COST	$7,950

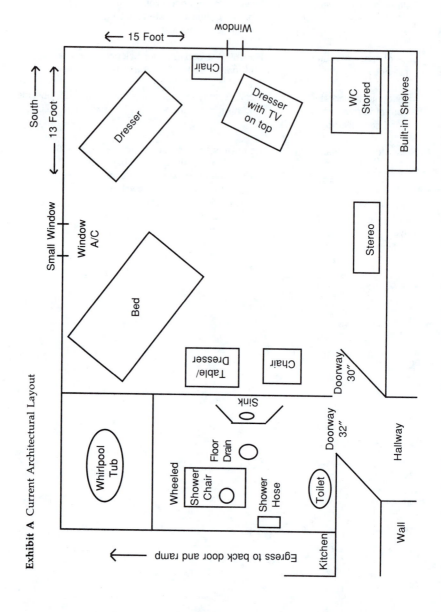

Exhibit A Current Architectural Layout

Exhibit B Suggested Architectural Layout

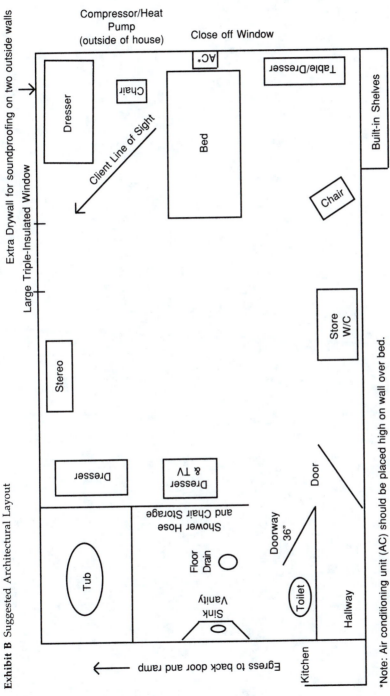

Appendix 4–C

Case Study #2: Rehabilitation Consultant's Report

Name: Martin Trent   **Date of report**: 2/1/95
DOB: 9/5/67
DOL: 11/16/81 & 12/14/93
Diagnoses: C4–5 quadriplegia   Autonomic disreflexia
Chronic pain and spasm   Neurogenic bladder
Frequent urinary tract infections   S/P burns to groin, with skin
Right ulnar neuropathy   grafting
                                          Temporal mandibular joint
                                             syndrome

Executive Summary

This report was generated at the request of the above-captioned patient's attorney. All available records were reviewed, and the patient was examined by a neurologist who saw him prior to the second accident and a neurosurgeon with expertise with traumatically injured patients.

Life Care Plan (see attachment)

The life care plan was constructed so as to give an estimate of the care requirements of Mr. Trent during his remaining estimated life to age 64. Past usage of equipment and supplies were taken into account to estimate future costs. Additional comments to the plan are as follows.

Medical Care and Hospitalizations

An estimate for the doctor visits is given, based on previous history. The patient did have one hospitalization for neurogenic bladder that caused him to have altered blood pressure that became life-threatening (autonomic dysflexia). A reasonable estimate for a recurrence of the autonomic dysreflexia or a severe urinary tract infection requiring hospitalization would be one every other year. Length of stay would probably be about four days. The present cost would be an estimated $7,500 per occurrence.

Nursing Care

Mr. Trent had his mother to care for him from the time of the first accident in 1981 until 9/2/94, when she became too ill to continue to assume those responsibilities. Although different prescriptions were written for six and eight hours of home health aides per day after discharge from Old South Rehabilitation Hospital in 1984, only two to four hours of home health nurses were used per day for six days per week. RN or LPN visits were done twice a day to catheterize the patient's bladder. With the mother home to attend to the patient's needs, and the additional home care services, it is reasonable to conclude that the patient would have needed 12 hours of nursing aide time per day before the second accident had the mother not been there. This is, in fact, what the neurologist estimated the care needs to be before the second accident.

The above care needs due to the first accident would have increased as the patient got older and his physical abilities decreased, as with any spinal-cord-injured person. Therefore, the level of care would have increased even if the second accident had not occurred.

The second accident caused the patient the loss of the ability to use his right arm and hand as he had previously. "This small change in function resulted in a major change in Mr. Trent's ability to be functional," as noted by Dr. Tourper in his report. Mr. Trent now also has markedly increased pain and muscle spasms of all his extremities. He complains of constant pain, which he rates 6 to 8 on a 10-point scale of severity. He is hesitant to take much pain medication because it causes drowsiness and does not work very well. He is now unable to care for himself or even shift the position of his body in bed.

Physical Therapy

An estimate of physical therapy expenses is given in order to maintain optimal function and thus decrease the possibility of expenses incurred due to decreased function, such as more pain, bladder and pulmonary infections, and pressure sores due to inactivity. Although the present treatment plans have not accounted for physical therapy "tune-ups," we feel that it would be money well spent.

Equipment

Van lift: Last purchased in 1991; usual life is 7 years. This would mean that this patient would require five more purchases of van lifts, at $3,500 installed.

Wheelchair: The electric wheelchair and seating system this patient now has is an Invacare Arrow with a layback system. This chair cost $20,000 but could have been purchased for much less had a rehab nurse been available to investigate alternatives. Additionally, this patient has had four chairs over the last 14 years, for an average life span of 3.5 years.

This is because of heavy use but also because the chairs were not periodically or properly maintained. In the past, Mr. Trent, Sr., maintained the chairs himself, charging only the cost of the spare parts to the insurance company. It is recommended that a service contract be arranged, with scheduled maintenance and a loaner chair planned, in order to extend the life of the chairs in the future.

Drugs

The cost estimates for the drugs used by the patient were made on the basis of past experience, but it is recommended that a mail-order service be engaged that will bring the cost of the drugs down and include overnight delivery. Computer flags of drug interactions and untoward effects are also recommended.

Medical Supplies

The cost of supplies to catheterize this patient is based on past experience, but there is no reason why this price cannot be moderated somewhat by a rehab nurse who can negotiate a better price.

Private Case Manager

The cost of hiring a private case manager for this patient is included in this life care plan as a cost-saving measure. Someone who is checking on the quality of services rendered and negotiating charges for equipment and pharmaceuticals will more than justify the estimated future cost of such a service.

Submitted by
Michael Newell, RN, MSN, CCM
Rehabilitation Consultant

Appendix 4–D

Case Study #2: Life Care Plan

Martin Trent: Present age 28; estimated life span, 64 years.

Care Needs	Purpose	Frequency	Costs	Future Costs
Medical treatment				
Physiatist	maintain optimal functioning	appointment every 3 months	$75/visit, $300/year	To be determined by economist
Urologist	treat urinary tract infections, bladder spasms	as needed, estimate 5 visits per year; urine cultures, estimate 5 per year	$75/visit, $375/year Urine cultures $80, $400/year	
General medical care	treat general medical conditions	as needed, estimate twice yearly	$40/visit, $80 yearly	
Psychologist	treatment of depression	once weekly	$80/visit, $4,160 yearly	
Hospitalizations	treatment of autonomic dysreflexia or urinary tract infections	estimate one every other year, more as patient grows older	$7,500 per occurrence, or $3,750 per year	
Nursing care				
Skilled	cath patient twice daily, supervise home health aides	14 visits per week	$80/visit, $58,400/year	
Unskilled	assistance with all activities of daily living, food preparation, transportation	24 hours per day	$16/hour, $385/day $140, 160/year; estimate half of total nursing costs attributable to accident of 12/6/80	
Physical therapy	maintain optimal function and range of motion of limbs	yearly "tune-up" for 6 weeks, 3 times per week	$60/visit, $1,080/year	
Equipment				
Van lift	access to van via wheelchair	daily use, replace every 7 years	$3,500 each, installed; $500/year	

Item	Description	Frequency	Cost
Wheelchair	self-locomotion	has been replaced every 3.5 years	$15,000 plus maintenance ($350/yr.), yearly cost approximately $4,635
Electric bed	assist with position in bed, prevent bedsores, and assist with patient's daily care routine	every 15 years	$1,580, yearly cost $105
Drugs			
Xylocaine 2% jelly	treat discomfort of daily catheterizations	33 tubes/year	@$22 = $726
Zoloft	treatment of depression	as prescribed	$245 in 1994
Valium	as needed for spasm	as needed	$213 in 1994
Procardia	spasm	as prescribed	$ 41 in 1994
Cipro	treat bladder infections	5 courses of treatment in 1994	$323 in 1994
Pain medication (Klonopin, Daypro)	analgesic, anti-flammatory	as prescribed	$ 90 in 1994
Medical supplies	urologicals: catheters, gloves, leg bags, catheter kits	cathed 2 to 4 times daily	$20,000 in 1994
Private case manager	coordinate care, especially payouts	review bills, care monthly	2 hours/month @$70/hr ($1,680/year)

Yearly costs: $237,140
Lifetime costs: $8,537,040

Submitted by

Michael Newell, RN, MSN, CCM

5

Professional Development of the Case Manager

Case managers are just beginning to gain an identity, thanks to the efforts of the Individual Case Management Association (ICMA), *The Case Manager* magazine, and the Case Management Society of America (CMSA). The CMSA is a nonprofit organization with a national structure and local chapters. Both organizations, along with an ad hoc group made up of individuals from the Insurance Rehabilitation Certification Commission, representatives from the American Nurses Association, the National Association of Rehabilitation Professionals in the Private Sector (NARPPS), and other case management organizations, came together to begin drawing up the process of standards and start a certification process in February 1991.[1]

Because case management has evolved from an insurance-payer perspective, involving little sharing of methods and almost no research for refereed journals in the area of medical (read nursing) case management, it has been hampered by a lack of common definitions and a common set of standards for education, ethical behavior, and practice.

The CMSA standards for the practice of case management indicate that the case manager should perform the functions of assessment; facilitation of communication to coordinate services; care planning and implementation, with the patient as the primary decision maker; and advocacy for the patient and client, while attempting to reach consensus between all parties. The case manager performs case identification and assessment, prob-

113

lem identification, planning, monitoring of the plan and process, and evaluation of services after the care is delivered. This includes an assessment of the outcomes and appropriateness of the care.

Standards-of-performance criteria in the CMSA proposal reiterate the need for quality services; collaboration; knowledge of and conformance with applicable federal and local laws; ethical behavior with respect to autonomy, dignity, and individual rights; and advocacy for the patient. Case managers are expected to refer, broker, or deliver services appropriate to the needs of the patient and the resources available. They are encouraged to develop new resources where there are gaps in the service continuum. They are expected to procure, monitor, coordinate, and evaluate services, as well as establish the eligibility and reimbursement of such services. Finally, they are expected to base their practice on research findings and to participate in research activity, including the collection of health outcomes data.

Appendix 5–B provides sample job descriptions for case manager positions in a variety of settings.

BACKGROUND AND TRAINING

The CMSA standards encourage a minimum of a baccalaureate degree or, in the case of a nurse, licensure and at least 24 months' experience in a job consisting of the above-described functions. Until recently, many nurse case managers entered the field through rehabilitation or home care. With the hospitals changing their internal practices, many nurses who had jobs in utilization review, discharge planning, quality assurance, risk management, or infectious disease are now directed to perform case management activity.

No set criteria are established to indicate who will do well as a case manager. Nurses who are resourceful problem solvers with a wide variety of clinical experience and good oral and written skills meet the minimum requirements to function successfully as case managers.

Individuals who are unable to abstract lessons from one setting to another, who are concrete thinkers, or who see their role as assisting the patient by doing or procuring extra services may not fit the expectations of the employers of case managers. Case managers must think "outside the box" because innovative solutions are required by the variety of complex situations that case managers are asked to address.

With the health system changing so rapidly, many nurses are looking at case management as a way to escape from the hospital setting, but they are discouraged by the requirements of previous experience, lower base pay, vague job descriptions, and (in many cases) scant training.

ASSESSING SUITABILITY FOR A CASE MANAGEMENT POSITION: TRANSFERABLE SKILLS ASSESSMENT

The skills necessary to be a case manager are not possessed by everyone. Those who are investigating the field may wish to fill out the following worksheets to discover which of their skills might be utilized in a case management setting. The process of analyzing transferable skills of claimants is somewhat similar.

Exhibits 5–1 through 5–4 are worksheets designed for use by nurses who want to find out what they do well and enjoy that might transfer to case management positions. (In some cases, case management may already be part of a current job but is not mentioned in the job title.) Exhibit 5–1 is designed to trigger a review of all the tasks and roles of current and past positions, including both those in which the nurse was successful and those that the nurse did *not* like doing or in which he or she rated him- or herself as not proficient. Exhibit 5–2 highlights skills and proficiences, including technical and people skills, acquired through formal and informal education, including self-improvement activities. Exhibit 5–3 is designed to highlight credentials, even those that may have been forgotten for a time.

Exhibit 5–4, the last worksheet, should enable the nurse to examine all skill sets discovered from the first three worksheets for transferability to case management. It asks the nurse to rephrase skills in terms of activities of *symbolic analysis.* This term comes from Robert Reich's book *The Work of Nations,*[2] which states that there are three basic types of work: routine production (such as manufacturing or clerical), in-person service (such as retail or restaurant), and symbolic analysis. Nursing seems to be a combination of the first two, in that most nurses are called upon to perform processes (technical and clerical) decided on by physicians, as well as to perform the physical caretaking functions that are expected by the public when they think of nursing.

Symbolic analysts are involved in problem identification and solving, brokering, negotiating fees, and finding the best value for others. They use information from a variety of sources to determine what course of action to take. Symbolic analysts know how systems operate, can abstract lessons and applications from one setting to another, and have a repertoire of techniques to bring to the complex problems that they are asked to solve. Symbolic analysts are also adept at collaborating with specialists in other disciplines and can function well when teamwork is called for. To become a case manager, one must move beyond the usual nursing roles of routine production and in-person service to become a symbolic analyst.

Taking our cue from Reich, we can conclude that case managers should be trained in systems thinking, collaboration, negotiation, and conflict

Exhibit 5–1 Case Management Transferable Skills Worksheet for Nurses: Work History

Start/Stop Dates of Work (Enter Most Recent Job First)	Name of Organization/Dept.	Description of All Duties or Activities	Responsibilities of Job, Fully or Partially (Be Expansive)	Successes: Things You Did Well and Enjoyed Doing	Limitations: Things You Did Not Do Well/Did Not Like

Exhibit 5–2 Case Management Transferable Skills Worksheet for Nurses: Educational Achievements (Formal and Informal Education, Including Self-Improvement)

Dates/Setting for Schooling or Training	Area of Concentration	Subjects of Projects, Articles, Presentations	Obstacles Encountered	Abilities or Skills Utilized in Overcoming Obstacles	Special Proficiencies Acquired, including Technical and People Skills

Exhibit 5–3 Case Management Transferable Skills Worksheet for Nurses: Formal Credentials

Credential or Special Recognition Received	Date Received/from Whom	Performance Required or Achievement Needed To Gain Recognition	Obstacles Overcome in the Course of Reaching Goal	Abilities Utilized To Overcome Obstacles Encountered	Proficiencies Demonstrated for Each Credential or Recognition

Exhibit 5–4 Case Management Transferable Skills Worksheet for Nurses: Transferable Skills Analysis

Enter Name or Description of Skills Identified in Previous Worksheets.	Specify the Subskills in Each Skill Entered in First Column. What Talents Are Evident?	Rephrase Skills and Talents in Terms of Activities Performed by Symbolic Analysts: (1) Problem Identification/Solving, (2) Information Finding/Systems, and (3) Negotiating/Coaching

resolution. They should have supervision support in terms of accessing medical, legal, and vocational information sources. They should also be conversant with outcomes measures that are relevant to the type of medical or vocational cases they are handling, including cost-benefit ratios for various proposed medical interventions and the case management intervention.

THE CASE MANAGER CERTIFICATION PROCESS

The case management certification exam is given twice a year by the Certification of Insurance Rehabilitation Specialists Commission.[3] This exam is quickly becoming the standard for ensuring that case managers have the experience to practice in the insurance setting. Internal case managers in hospitals may find the exam difficult because of the emphasis on insurance systems and rehabilitation issues. Appendix 5–C lists topics covered in the certification exam for case managers. Most of these topics are covered throughout this book.

NOTES

1. Case Management Society of America, CMSA Proposes Standards of Practice, *The Case Manager* 5, no. 1 (1994):59–70.
2. R. Reich, *The Work of Nations* (New York: Knopf, 1994).
3. Certification of Insurance Rehabilitation Specialists Commission, 1835 Rowling Road, Suite D, Rolling Meadows, IL 60008, phone (708) 818-0292.

Appendix 5–A

Job Descriptions for Long-Term Care Facility

The following job descriptions were written for a long-term care facility that was adopting a case management model. These job descriptions address issues of all skilled nursing facilities and were written to redefine the roles of the hands-on caregivers. The role of the case manager is defined as focusing on the patient, not adding an extra level of formal supervision to the staff. The job descriptions of the charge nurse and nursing assistant were rewritten so as to support the patient-focused aspects of the case management model and to more clearly delineate their roles at a time when the expectations of the care at the facility (and at all skilled nursing and long-term care facilities) are rising secondary to public and regulatory expectations. The following job descriptions were composed to facilitate performance appraisals, and were posted for all to read so that each team member would be aware of his or her change in roles.

NURSE CASE MANAGER

Name: _____   Date: _____

Evaluator Name:_____

Scoring Legend: 5. Consistently exceeds standard
4. Occasionally exceeds standard
3. Consistently meets standard
2. Occasionally meets standards
1. Consistently does not meet standard

I. UNIVERSAL STANDARDS

	5	4	3	2	1
A. Demonstrates professionalism and sensitivity when interacting with residents, families, and coworkers. Creates and maintains an environment conducive to teamwork. Upholds appropriate levels of confidentiality and discretion. Maintains respect for residents' rights.	()	()	()	()	()
B. Dresses in a way that enhances the professional role of the case manager.	()	()	()	()	()

C. Arrives at work at scheduled starting time.   () () () () ()
Demonstrates reasonable effort to attend
meetings in a timely manner.

D. Is conscious and aware of environmental factors   () () () () ()
that may pose a safety hazard to residents
and employees. Takes the necessary
precautions and preventive measures to
ensure a safe atmosphere. Reports and acts
on reports of others regarding incidents of
injury or abuse.

E. Functions within the professional nursing law   () () () () ()
and the ANA code of ethics.

F. Reports and documents when nursing standards   () () () () ()
of care are not upheld.

G. Recognizes areas of professional limitations and   () () () () ()
seeks opportunities for growth by
attending educational offerings relevant to
needs.

H. Actively participates in student education   () () () () ()
programs when in place.

I. Actively involved in Quality Assurance Process.   () () () () ()

II. COORDINATION OF RESIDENT CARE

A. Assessment

   1. Performs initial assessment and   () () () () ()
      documents data systematically from all
      sources.

   2. Performs ongoing assessments documenting   () () () () ()
      resident status and needs.

   3. Demonstrates expertise in integrating   () () () () ()
      physical, social, and psychological data
      to make a realistic assessment.

   4. Utilizes appropriate verbal and nonverbal   () () () () ()
      interviewing skills to ascertain care
      needs.

   5. Monitors appropriate use of and   () () () () ()
      documentation concerning physical
      restraints.

   6. Monitors use of psychotropic medications   () () () () ()
      for appropriateness and side effects.
      Documents assessments on three-

month summary and performs AMES
test when indicated.

7. Monitors nutrition and hydration status,   () () () () ()
including weight gains or losses, and
documents appropriate intervention
steps.

8. Assesses the need for other resources (e.g.,   () () () () ()
therapists, consultants, counselors) and
initiates appropriate use of resources.

B. Diagnosis and Classification

1. Formulates an appropriate nursing   () () () () ()
diagnosis based on analysis of the
database.

2. Evidences an understanding of the MDS and   () () () () ()
RAPs system of patient classification by
making such patient classifications
according to established criteria.
Follows up on changes in classification.

C. Planning

1. Formulates a realistic, goal-oriented nursing   () () () () ()
care plan based on the nursing
diagnosis and classification tools.

2. Maintains a current and comprehensive care   () () () () ()
plan based on continuing assessments
of the resident's status.

3. Writes individualized interventions and   () () () () ()
parameters with instructions that are
appropriate to the achievement of the
goals.

4. Contracts with the resident and all appropriate   () () () () ()
parties to carry out the care plan.

5. Documents resident and family involvement   () () () () ()
and understanding of care plan and
contract.

6. Documents progress toward attainment of   () () () () ()
goals and outcomes of interventions in
reference to the care plan.

7. Documents involvement of other health   () () () () ()
care team members in setting and
carrying out realistic goals for the
resident. Attends care planning
meetings.

D. Implementation
  1. Action
     a. Initiates and demonstrates knowledge   () () () () ()
        of the case management process
        through utilization of appropriate
        interventions and documentation of
        same.
     b. Ensures that nursing care is delivered in   () () () () ()
        accordance with established policies
        and procedures.
     c. Ensures that nursing care is delivered with () () () () ()
        the appropriate frequency of
        duration to address resident care
        needs.
     d. Follows established protocol with regard   () () () () ()
        to infection control issues (e.g., hand
        washing, disposing) and maintains a
        correct and appropriate level of
        documentation regarding each
        incident in which infection control
        procedure is used.
     e. Discusses advance directives and living   () () () () ()
        will issues with residents, families,
        and all interested parties to ensure
        that the resident's wishes are
        pursued with respect to medical
        interventions.
     f. Utilizes community and facility resouces   () () () () ()
        appropriately.
  2. Plan of Treatment
     a. Integrates plan of treatment with ongoing   () () () () ()
        resident care activities.
     b. Utilizes sound nursing judgment in   () () () () ()
        implementing therapeutic regime.
  3. Documentation
     a. Utilizes the correct forms to document   () () () () ()
        patient status, plan of care, and
        ongoing changes.
     b. Records new orders in resident chart in   () () () () ()
        accordance with established protocol.
     c. Ensures that records are complete, concise, () () () () ()
        accurate, legible, dated, and signed.

4. Interdisciplinary
   a. Delegates personal care activities to   () () () () ()
      licensed and certified nursing
      personnel.
   b. Shares in the supervision of the above   () () () () ()
      caregivers by use of negotiation.
      Provides documentation concerning
      the skill levels, cooperation, and
      level of care observed.
   c. Confers with all disciplines involved in the   () () () () ()
      care of the residents.
   d. Reports changes in clinical status to clinical () () () () ()
      supervisors, physicians, and other
      members of the health care team.
   e. Communicates important aspects of   () () () () ()
      resident care whenever case
      manager is unavailable to carry out
      the care plan.
5. Teaching
   a. Provides verbal instructions,   () () () () ()
      demonstrations, and written
      materials to residents, families, and
      other team members.
   b. Utilizes available resources to aid in   () () () () ()
      teaching.
   c. Discusses care and specific treatment   () () () () ()
      modalities to receive resident/
      guardian's consent and
      understanding prior to the initiation
      of care.
   d. Educates resident, family, and other team   () () () () ()
      members on the therapeutic action,
      side effects, dosage, etc., of
      medications.
E. Evaluation
   1. Documents the effectiveness of nursing   () () () () ()
      care and progress toward goal attainment.
   2. Modifies the plan of care in a timely fashion.   () () () () ()
   3. Collaborates with other team members to   () () () () ()
      determine the effectiveness of
      prescribed treatment and resident
      response.

4. Participates in facility quality assurance efforts or other designated monitoring programs.   () () () () ()

5. Evaluates all equipment in use with resident in reference to appropriateness and proper functioning. Initiates changes as necessary.   () () () () ()

III. PROFESSIONAL/PERSONAL RESPONSIBILITY AND GROWTH

A. Maintains an acceptable level of productivity.   () () () () ()

B. Follows accepted procedure for requesting benefit time. Prepares sign-off regarding caseload.   () () () () ()

C. Attends and participates in training sessions.   () () () () ()

D. Follows established lines of communications and authority.   () () () () ()

E. Completes agency forms as per protocol and submits on a timely basis (i.e., assessment forms, care plans, daily contact sheets, classification forms, etc.).   () () () () ()

CHARGE NURSE (RN or LPN)

Name: _____ Date: _____

Evaluator Name: _____

Scoring Legend: 5. Consistently exceeds standard
4. Occasionally exceeds standard
3. Consistently meets standard
2. Occasionally meets standards
1. Consistently does not meet standard

I. UNIVERSAL STANDARDS

	5	4	3	2	1
A. Demonstrates professionalism and sensitivity when interacting with residents, families, and coworkers. Actively participates in the treatment team. Maintains confidentiality and discretion. Maintains respect for residents' and coworkers' rights.	()	()	()	()	()
B. Dress is standard white, making a neat appearance. Dress style will promote efficient hygiene. Dress accessories will not cause a safety hazard to the resident or the nurse.	()	()	()	()	()
C. Arrives at work at scheduled starting time. Attends scheduled meetings in a timely manner.	()	()	()	()	()
D. Takes reasonable precautions that will promote safety in the workplace for both residents and coworkers. Reports and acts on the reports of others regarding issues of injury or abuse.	()	()	()	()	()
E. Functions within nursing laws and the policies of the facility.	()	()	()	()	()
F. Reports and documents when nursing standards of care are not upheld.	()	()	()	()	()

G. Demonstrates reasonable effort to increase skill   ()   ()   ()   () ()
    level and adapt to new expectations in
    terms of job performance.

H. Actively participates in student education   ()   ()   ()   () ()
    programs when in place.

II. STANDARD OF RESIDENT CARE

A. Assessment
  1. Observes patients and does assessments   ()   ()   ()   () ()
     in the course of duties. Acts on the
     information of others with regard to
     following up on assessments. Assesses
     residents' responses to treatment plans.
  2. Effectively communicates to superiors and   ()   ()   ()   () ()
     subordinates any changes in resident
     health status. Documents accurate
     assessments.
  3. Assesses assignments of nursing care of   ()   ()   ()   () ()
     residents, makes assignments in a fair
     and timely fashion.
  4. Assesses level of nursing care administered to   ()   ()   ()   () ()
     residents by nursing assistants and
     other nursing personnel. Documents
     superior care as well as deficiencies.

B. Communication
  1. Communicates relevant information during   ()   ()   ()   () ()
     shift report and passes on information
     to team members in a timely fashion.
  2. Documents relevant information in the proper   ()   ()   ()   () ()
     formats concerning assessments,
     interventions, progress of care, and
     unusual incidents regarding nursing
     care administered to residents.
  3. Functions as an integral health team member,   ()   ()   ()   () ()
     coordinating direct nursing care and
     response to care.
  4. Under the supervision and support of the   ()   ()   ()   () ()
     nursing supervisor, gives relevant
     information to team members and
     subordinates regarding quality of care
     delivered.

C. Planning
  1. Participates in developing the plan of care and   () () () () ()
     takes responsibility to ensure that
     nursing care plans are carried out.
  2. Provides documentation regarding the   () () () () ()
     response to the plan of care.
  3. Plans resource use regarding maintenance   () () () () ()
     of nursing care. This includes directing
     personnel, supplies, equipment, and
     other resources.
  4. Revises resident care plans in accordance with   () () () () ()
     changes in the residents' status.
D. Implementation
  1. Passes medication using safe procedures,   () () () () ()
     including knowledge of adverse
     reactions.
  2. Documents in a clear, legible fashion. Verbally   () () () () ()
     communicates in an effective and
     appropriate manner.
  3. Performs skilled treatments properly and as   () () () () ()
     ordered.
  4. Follows established protocol regarding   () () () () ()
     infection control issues. Demonstrates
     understanding of infection control
     issues.
E. Evaluation
  1. Evaluates the care of subordinates and   () () () () ()
     provides rationales for such
     evaluations.
  2. Observes resident responses to care rendered   () () () () ()
     or daily events. Communicates relevant
     observations to case manager and other
     team members.
  3. Collaborates with other team members to   () () () () ()
     determine the effectiveness of
     prescribed treatment and resident
     response.
  4. Promptly reports any malfunctioning or unsafe   () () () () ()
     equipment.
  5. Records relevant observations on an as-needed   () () () () ()
     basis.

CERTIFIED NURSING ASSISTANT

Name: _____   Date: _____

Evaluator Name:_____

Scoring Legend: 5. Consistently exceeds standard
4. Occasionally exceeds standard
3. Consistently meets standard
2. Occasionally meets standards
1. Consistently does not meet standard

I. UNIVERSAL STANDARDS

	5	4	3	2	1
A. Demonstrates professionalism and sensitivity when interacting with residents, families, and coworkers. Actively participates on the treatment team. Maintains confidentiality and discretion. Maintains respect for residents' and coworkers' rights.	()	()	()	()	()
B. Dress is standard white, making a neat appearance. Dress style will promote hygiene, and accessories will not cause a safety hazard to the resident or the nursing assistant.	()	()	()	()	()
C. Arrives at work at scheduled starting time. Attends scheduled meetings in a timely manner.	()	()	()	()	()
D. Takes reasonable precautions that will promote safety in the workplace for both residents and coworkers. Reports and acts on the reports of others regarding issues of abuse.	()	()	()	()	()
E. Functions within the policies of the facility.	()	()	()	()	()
F. Reports and documents nursing care.	()	()	()	()	()
G. Demonstrates reasonable effort to increase skill level and adapt to new expectations of job performance.	()	()	()	()	()

II. STANDARD OF RESIDENT CARE

A. Assessment

1. Assesses general condition of the patient at the   ()   ()   ()   () () beginning of each shift and accepts the care of each patient with knowledge of what the treatment plan is.

2. Communicates any change in patient status   ()   ()   ()   () () in a timely fashion to the charge nurse or nursing supervisor. Makes relevant facts known.

3. Demonstrates proficiency or willingness   ()   ()   ()   () () to seek proficiency in diagnostic skills related to vital signs and physical assessments.

B. Planning

1. Makes observations known or otherwise   ()   ()   ()   () () participates in planning sessions or conferences related to planning resident care.

2. Is aware of resident's current treatment plan   ()   ()   ()   () () and suggests modifications as needed.

3. Plans own workload so as to effectively   ()   ()   ()   () () complete assignments within a reasonable time frame.

4. Plans personal time well in advance so that   ()   ()   ()   () () suitable efforts can be made to account for unit staffing.

C. Implementation

1. Administers skilled nursing care to residents,   ()   ()   ()   () () demonstrating a high standard of care in the areas of nutrition, hygiene, safety, skin care, and emotional support.

2. Carries out the treatment plan for assigned   ()   ()   ()   () () residents, including toileting, ambulation, feeding, positioning, and range-of-motion exercises.

3. Interacts with residents in a respectful and   ()   ()   ()   () () therapeutic manner.

    4. Maintains good standard of practice when   ()   ()   ()   () ()
       involved in isolation and other
       infectious disease issues.

D. Evaluation

    1. Observes resident response to care rendered   ()   ()   ()   () ()
       or daily events. Communicates relevant
       observations to charge nurse, case
       manager, and other team members.

    2. Collaborates with other team   ()   ()   ()   () ()
       members to determine the effectiveness
       of prescribed treatment and resident
       response.

    3. Promptly reports any malfunctioning or unsafe ()   ()   ()   () ()
       equipment.

    4. Records relevant observations on an as-needed ()   ()   ()   () ()
       basis.

Appendix 5-B

Sample Case Manager Job Descriptions

INTERNAL CASE MANAGER: SUBACUTE CARE CENTER (PART OF A LONG-TERM CARE FACILITY)

Reports to: Subacute Program Director

Major objectives of position:

1. Coordinate all patient admissions from point of possible referral through discharge.
2. Be a liaison to the referral source/payer.
3. Coordinate care of patients while they are in the subacute program.
4. Assist in marketing subacute care program.

Qualifications:

B.S.N., five years' nursing experience, preferably in rehabilitation, case management, trauma care, and/or equivalent activity. Good oral and written communication skills, including public speaking. Ability to use word processor. Certification as case manager (CCM) or as a rehabilitation nurse (CRRN), or qualified to sit for exam and obtain certification within one year of employment.

Major responsibilities:

1. Coordinate insurance-related preadmission, including verification of coverage and benefits, negotiation of rate, and securing a letter of agreement for admission.
2. Travel to see patient and conduct a preadmission evaluation to determine level of care required and appropriateness of admission to subacute facility.
3. Coordinate and implement care plan once admission to facility occurs. Communicate care plan to payer case manager, communicate changes in patient status or intensiveness of service, and plan discharge.
4. Handle reimbursement issues, including obtaining prior authorization for changes in intensiveness of service or care plan.
5. Conduct weekly team meetings/care plan meetings regarding patients being case managed.

6. Coordinate with quality improvement coordinator the following: clinical, financial, and patient satisfaction outcomes data. Report data and recommendations to program director.
7. Plan and conduct training for facility staff regarding clinical issues important to subacute program. Plan and coordinate with director of marketing one seminar for referral sources/case managers each year.
8. Conduct marketing activity that enhances the reputation and visibility of the subacute program at the direction of the marketing director.
9. Demonstrate a professional demeanor in appearance and all aspects of communication within and outside of the facility.

EXTERNAL UTILIZATION REVIEW COORDINATOR

Reports to: Branch Manager

Major objectives of position:

1. Prescreen provider invoices to determine whether they should be reviewed further, using automated bill review product or full review with records.
2. Review provider bills to determine if the bills fulfill requirements for full reimbursement. The criteria in question include procedure codes congruent with diagnosis, medical necessity, appropriate level of charge or intensiveness of service, and acceptable medical practice.
3. Enhance the ability of the company to maximize savings to the client.

Qualifications:

Five years' nursing experience, preferably in emergency room, orthopedics, occupational health, or rehabilition. Prior utilization review experiences preferred. Good oral and written communication skills. Facility with state workers' compensation law.

Job responsibilities:

1. Review medical bills for correct coding, relationship of service to the covered injury, and relation of the charge to the fee schedule or usual and customary charge, depending on the type of coverage.
2. Review medical records and documentation to support provider charges.
3. Serve as an authoritative resource for other branch personnel regarding clinical interpretation of medical or rehabilitation procedures.
4. Conduct in-service training as directed by branch manager for all staff regarding clinical practices, billing practices, and changes in the CPT coding manual and practice as they relate to the use of modifiers and other documentation to support the provider bill or claim.
5. Respond to all client inquiries regarding billing practices or claims review.
6. Respond to all provider requests for reconsideration of payment levels within the legal mandate for reconsideration requests (varies by state).

7. Review and validate written provider requests for clarification or additional payment.
8. Negotiate payment of claims with providers based on information gathered in review.
9. Instruct data entry personnel regarding unusual bills that may need clarification as to category before being input for automated bill review.
10. Act as a resource for marketing personnel on as-needed basis to explain services of the company.

UNIT-BASED ACUTE CARE CASE MANAGER

Reports to: Director of Case Management

Major objectives of the position:

1. Perform utilization review, risk management, discharge planning, and patient education on a 32-bed surgical nursing unit.
2. Guide the development of critical paths for selected sets of patients in conjunction with medical staff and quality improvement teams.
3. This position has no "hands-on" patient contact responsibilities, but is intended to enhance and coordinate the communication between the treatment team, the patient/family, and the payer sources.

Qualifications:

B.S.N., five years of progressive experience, preferably in one of the following areas: utilization review, risk management, discharge planning, quality assurance.

Job responsibilities:

1. Identify high-risk patients on admission to the hospital in conjunction with the nursing assessment done by staff nurses.
2. Identify length-of-stay parameters by dianosis with all high-risk patients.
3. Participate in the a.m. and p.m. shift reports daily. Communicate issues regarding selected patients to team members.
4. Review documentation or use of critical-path flowcharts on case-managed patients for quality of documentation and the ability of flowcharts to reflect patient status accurately. Review outlier incidents and patients so as to resolve difficulties.
5. Communicate with physicians, families, payer sources, and follow-up care providers regarding patient status and progress, anticipated length of stay, expected functional outcome of care, and discharge requirements.
6. Identify patient/family teaching needs so as to facilitate optimal discharge.
7. Revise policies, procedures, and protocols on nursing unit in conjunction with head nurse and case management supervisor.

8. Mediate disputes between nursing and other departments regarding duties and responsibilities, breakdowns in quality, and patient/family complaints.
9. Collect process data and clinical outcome data as directed by the QI team.
10. Train and implement critical pathways for unit as they become available. Follow up to ensure that pathways and documentation are complete. Take complaints/suggestions for changes back to the QI team as necessary.
11. Conduct unit-specific training programs for staff as necessary.
12. Document variances from critical paths or patient outcomes regarding health status, length of stay, or iatrogenic incidents. Prepare monthly report for case management supervisor and QI team.
13. Investigate all incidents involving patients and make recommendations to head nurse and risk manager within one week of incident.

MEDICAL CASE MANAGER FOR INDEPENDENT CASE MANAGEMENT COMPANY

Reports to: Office Manager

Major objectives of position:

1. Conduct medical assessment and case management of client referrals.
2. Draw up return-to-work plans for claimants to return to original employer.
3. Promote effective business relationships with business clients so as to enhance case referrals.

Qualifications:

RN with five or more years of experience, preferably in case management, rehabilitation, orthopedics, or utilization review. Good oral and written communication skills. CCM or CRRN preferred.

Job responsibilities:

1. Perform initial assessment of the claimant on site within five business days of referral, where possible.
2. Propose rehabilitation action plan and recommendations so as to facilitate recovery and return to work within state workers' compensation statute and customer guidelines.
3. Work with attending physician and other providers to coordinate and facilitate treatment for the claimant.
4. Communicate to referral source as needed, and make a written report at least every 30 days.
5. Document all case activity in progress reports and case notes.
6. Provide support to claimant and family as needed.
7. Interact with union representative, legal representative, shop foreman, personnel director, etc., in an assertive, influential manner.
8. Obtain signed job description and functional capacity assessments from attending physician or IME consultants.

9. Perform transferable skills assessments, career guidance, and counseling where appropriate.
10. Provide cost projections and cost-benefit analysis of treatment options and case management activity.
11. Provide marketing support for account executive regarding specific capabilities of case management activity.

Appendix 5–C

Topics on the
Case Management
Certification Exam

TOPICS ON THE CASE MANAGEMENT
CERTIFICATION EXAM

1. when/how/why cost-benefit analysis
2. coverage/exclusions/conditions of types of insurance policies
3. eligibility criteria for funding sources in public and private sectors
4. procedures to negotiate extracontractual coverage
5. philosophy of workers' compensation systems
6. how to evaluate appropriateness of medical care
7. how to identify cases that are high risk for complications
8. case management philosophies and principles
9. standards of case management
10. liability issues for case managers
11. care-planning and goal development techniques
12. principles of self-determination and empowerment
13. psychological effects of disabling conditions
14. ethical principles in the case management process
15. alternative funding sources in the public sector
16. the Americans with Disabilities Act (ADA)
17. the Individuals with Disabilities Education Act (IDEA)
18. principles of disability management
19. principles of informed consent
20. methodology for establishing transferable skills in vocational reha-bilitation
21. philosophy of hospice and palliative care
22. the deposition process
23. legal terminology
24. insurance terminology and contracts
25. general principles and philosophy of rehabilitation

Part II

Engaging the
Patient

⟨❦⟩

6

From Quality Assurance to Quality Improvement

One of the most difficult transitions that health clinicians have had to struggle with over the last few years has been the shift from *quality assurance* (QA) to *quality improvement* (QI; a term understood here to include *continuous quality improvement, total quality management,* and the Joint Commission's latest term *process improvement*). In general, QA focuses on reducing errors, meeting standards set up by the provider organization or by external licensing and other regulatory bodies, and measuring provider-defined outcomes. It works episodically, in response to problems, and retrospectively, tracking outliers and determining accountability once errors have occurred. QI, in contrast, focuses on improving processes, meeting the needs of the customer, and measuring customer-defined outcomes. It works continuously and proactively and involves all employees in the activities of systems evaluation and systems change.

The purpose of this chapter is to:

1. review how QA and QI have been implemented in the health care field
2. examine the limitations of QA and its measures and the causes of the transition to a QI paradigm
3. explore the connections between QI and case mangement
4. examine QI measures of health outcomes and show how they can be used by case managers

5. explore the link between health outcomes and health-related quality of life

QA IN HEALTH CARE

History of QA

QA in health care began in the nineteenth century when Florence Nightingale began gathering and disseminating statistics on mortality in hospitals. It was continued in the early 1900s by Ernest Codman, whose attempts to determine the quality of surgical care by linking morbidity and mortality to surgical intervention and errors led to the establishment, by the American College of Surgeons in 1913, of a Hospital Standardization Program to ensure that minimum standards of care were met (see Table 6–1 for a summary of major events in hospital quality management).

In 1951, the Joint Commission on Accreditation of Healthcare Organizations was established. It and other accrediting and licensing bodies originally focused on *structural measures* of quality: the physical plant, number of nurses per bed, the credentials of physicians and other service providers, and the presence of a set of standards by which departments and individuals would be held accountable. They used a system of inspection to evaluate conformance to standards, but they did not evaluate the actual quality of care delivered, and the structural features that they required were not necessarily indicators of quality.[1] Nor did they investigate causation or fault if there was a quality problem.

In 1966, Donabedian introduced a framework for rethinking the delivery of quality medical services.[2] He categorized three types of quality measures: structural, process, and outcomes (examples are listed in Table 6–2). In the ensuing decades, his model would prove influential in shifting attention from structure to process and outcome indicators. The Professional Standards Review Organization (PSRO), created for review of QA and utilization in 1972, placed little emphasis on structural indicators but a strong emphasis on the process of medical care delivery by physicians.

In 1979, the Joint Commission changed its procedures from requiring a preset number of audits to taking a problem-oriented approach. The problem-oriented approach dictated that hospitals gather data on unexpected or adverse occurrences. Mortality rates outside of predictions (outliers), falls, urinary tract infections, and various iatrogenic events were supposed to be identified. The QA committees were then supposed to show that steps were taken to correct these problems.

In response to this development, hospitals set up QA committees to review problem areas. Futher, during the 1980s, external (to the hospital)

physician peer review organizations (PROs) and utilization review companies with worker's compensation, auto insurance carriers, and third-party administrators attempted to provide some oversight of quality. But all these systems were hampered by hospital cultures that too often protected the rights of physician providers while ensuring only minimal compliance, on paper, with practice standards. And the retrospective and standards-oriented QA system proved to be inherently unfair and inefficient. Retrospective chart/utilization review was expensive, and after-the-fact reviews reflected more how the paperwork looked than how the patient fared. Risk management methodologies did improve, but not enough to stem the increase in jury awards for malpractice claims or to meet the rising consumer expectations regarding the quality of care to be delivered. In 1989, the Institute of Medicine concluded that "systematic evidence of the impact of utilization management methods on the quality of care or on patient and provider costs is virtually nonexistent."[3] And in 1990, one commentator in *Health Care Management Review* stated:

> A cynical description of today's state of affairs is that punitive, witch-hunting regulators vainly attempt to inspect an entrenched clan of professionals who protect, but do not discipline, each other despite delivering inadequate or inappropriate services to customers who cannot tell what they are getting for ever-increasing prices.[4]

QA Outcomes Measures

As indicated earlier, QA in the health field has a long tradition of measuring quality by mortality and morbidity statistics. *Mortality* is the death rate per admissions to a hospital; it can also be determined in relation to other populations, such as a diagnostic category, a treatment category, or covered lives. *Morbidity* is the rate of unforeseen events that occur secondary to a medical intervention, causing decline in patient health or functional ability—for example, hospital-acquired infections, surgical complications, and falls.

Both mortality and morbidity are affected by patient characteristics, such as age, severity of principal diagnosis, severity and extent of comorbidities, functional status, socioeconomic status, and even the attitude that the patient brings to the intervention. (See Exhibit 6–1). Florence Nightingale, although she instituted the collection of such statistics, criticized their use because of the difficulty of getting valid information on such factors as health prior to admission.[5] Today most mortality statistics

Table 6–1 Evolution of Hospital Quality Management

Time Line	Major Events	Impact on Hospitals' Structures
Early to mid-1900s	Components of Codman's "end result" idea are incorporated into the founding of the American College of Surgeons in 1913, its adoption of the minimum standard and the Hospital Standardization Program.	
1951	Joint Commission on Accreditation of Hospitals established.	
1960s	Landmark case of *Darling v. Charleston Community Memorial Hospital* (1965); Donabedian's formulation of structure, process, and outcome approaches to the assessment of quality (1966).	Begin to have dedicated staff involved with quality assurance and risk management.
1970s	Public Law 92-603 creates the Professional Standards Review Organization (PSRO) for review of quality assurance and utilization in 1972.	Dedicated staff and departments for quality assurance in response to accreditation demands, utilization review in response to the PSRO requirements, and risk management in response to increased malpractice claims. Also, formed committees to address these functions.
	Joint Commission begins to require a preset number of audits in 1975, replaced by a problem-oriented approach in the first quality assurance standard of 1979.	
Early to mid-1980s	Utilization Review: The number of reviews increase as PSROs change to peer review organizations for the Medicare program and prospective payment methods are embraced by many reimbursers.	Increases in utilization review staff.
	Risk Management: (1) Case-finding methods proliferate and (2) jury settlements escalate, accompanied by increased malpractice premiums, withdrawal of insurance companies from some markets, and abandonment of physician's practices.	Increases in risk management staff—specifically, increased number of positions for in-house legal counsel.

Table 6–1 continued

Time Line	Major Events	Impact on Hospitals' Structures
	Quality Assurance: Joint Commission changes to ongoing monitoring and evaluation for clinical services: increased emphasis on the role of the governing board in overseeing quality.	Increases in staff devoted to quality assurance.
Late 1980s to present	1. Conceptual links established between quality and risk management, and quality assurance and utilization review in Donabedian's discussions of provider-client-level quality.	More interaction between staff in quality assurance, utilization management, risk management, medical staff office, medical records, and information systems, leading to some departmental consolidations.
	2. Joint Commission develops 10-step process.	
	3. Initiatives dependent on large databases for case-mix- and severity-adjustment systems and outcomes research introduced.	
	4. Continuous quality improvement introduced.	

Source: Reprinted from Genevich-Richards, J., Quality Management Organizational Structure: History and Trend, *Journal for Healthcare Quality*, Vol. 16, No. 1, p. 23, with permission of the National Association for Healthcare Quality, 5700 Old Orchard Road, First Floor, Skokie, IL 60077-1057. Copyright © 1994, National Association for Healthcare Quality.

are judged in relation to an expected norm, usually based on a severity index. Severity indices are concurrently or retrospectively abstracted variances from the expected clinical norm, or are risk adjusted using covariances.[6] Morbidity rates can also be to some extent risk adjusted. But at best, mortality and morbidity statistics provide a gross, overgeneralized, and not very useful measure of the quality of a facility's services. Further, the procedures for use of outcomes data that take into account a facility's case-mix adjustment have not yet been standardized, so that meaningful comparisons among facilities are generally not possible.[7]

A third group of QA measures, *clinical status* measures, includes objective biochemical, physiological, anatomical, and histological indicators of disease, such as presenting signs or the results of laboratory tests or x-rays.

Table 6–2 Donabedian's Structure-Process-Outcomes Framework for Quality Indicators in Health Care

Structure Indicators	Process Indicators	Outcomes Indicators
System Characteristics: organization specialty mix financial incentives workload access/convenience	Administrative: admissions ancillary services information systems medical records nursing support	Clinical Endpoints: signs and symptoms lab values death
Institutional Characteristics: location physical plant nurses/bed equipment	Technical Style: visits medications referrals test ordering hospitalizations	Functional Status: physical mental social role
Provider Characteristics: age gender specialty training economic incentives beliefs/attitudes job satisfaction	resources utilization coordination/continuity Interpersonal Style: communication level patient participation teaching/counseling interpersonal "fit"	General Well-Being: health perceptions energy/fatigue pain life satisfaction
Patient Characteristics: age gender diagnosis/condition severity comorbidity beliefs/attitudes health habits preferences		Satisfaction with Care: access convenience cost perception of quality

Source: Adapted from Tarlov, A.R., et al., The Medical Outcomes Study: An Application of Methods for Monitoring the Results of Medical Care, *Journal of the American Medical Association*, Vol. 262, No. 7, p. 926, with permission of the American Medical Association, © 1989.

Such measures have traditionally been the "hard data" by which the efficiency and efficacy of care has been judged, and they are the indices that physicians have been trained and socialized to use in guiding and evaluating care.

Yet the medical literature is replete with structural findings (radiographic, laboratory, MRI, etc.) that have little correlation to clinical and/or

Exhibit 6–1 Types of Comorbid Conditions

- Age
- Sex
- Acute clinical stability
- Principal diagnosis ("case mix")
- Severity of principle diagnosis
- Extent and severity of comorbidities
- Physical functional status
- Psychological, cognitive and psychosocial functioning
- Cultural, ethnic, and socioeconomic attributes and behaviors
- Health status and quality of life
- Patient attitudes and preferences for outcomes

Source: Compiled from Iezzoni, L.I., Dimensions of Risk, in *Risk Adjustment for Measuring Health Care Outcomes*, p. 31, Health Administration Press, 1994.

functional health.[8] "The reliability of many signs, procedures and diagnostic and therapeutic judgments has never been studied. . . . Moreover, physicians' judgments regarding the quality of care may only be weakly related to the outcomes of care."[9] A patient can have a poor cardiac output as measured by an echocardiograph, yet be able to assume all the duties that his or her role in life demands. Snellen eye chart data may indicate acceptable visual acuity but may not correlate with functional visual status.

The pursuit of a "gold standard" for assessing quality in the provision of health services has not worked because the biologic aspect is only one aspect of the person. Disease is a biopsychosocial phenomenon that is not amenable to one-dimensional standards. Thus, although clinical measures can yield inferences or clues concerning the patient's condition, as outcome measures, they may give little useful information concerning patient-defined and societally defined utilities.

QA outcomes measures are summarized with examples in Table 6–3.

THE SHIFT FROM QA TO QI

In 1992 the Joint Commission, in its *Accreditation Manual for Hospitals*, announced its adoption of new standards designed to reorient health providers (in that these standards are now reflected in all other standards manuals: rehab, subacute, long-term care and home care) to continuous

Table 6–3 QA Outcomes Measures

Outcome Measure	Definition	Examples
Mortality	number of deaths observed vs. number expected, adjusted for risk factors	percentage of coronary bypass surgery deaths adjusted for age and other risk factors
Morbidity	an unforeseen event that occurs secondary to a medical intervention, causing decline in patient health or functional ability	hospital acquired infections, surgical misadventures, falls
Clinical outcome	traditional measures used by doctors to measure patient status	controlled blood glucose for a diabetic, survival for >5 years for a cancer patient

quality improvement.[10] The concepts and practices of QI had been introduced into American industry by W.E. Deming and Joseph Juran in the 1980s.

Juran defined *quality* as "product features which meet customer needs" —that is, conformance to customer specifications and fitness for use.[11] Quality, then, was defined not by the providers but by the customers— whether these were external (e.g., clients, buyers, government regulators), internal (e.g., employees, key suppliers, stockholders, and others with an interest in the company's doing well), or users (e.g., resellers, service entities, consumers, and other end users).

A critical issue with respect to quality is the number of "re-dos" that a provider must carry out to satisfy the customer. A re-do is anything that has to be done over because it did not meet required specifications the first time. Juran claimed that 15 to 25 percent of the cost of doing business is typically re-dos and that most of this chronic waste is due to poor planning. Juran further postulated that the cost of good quality is *less than* the cost of poor quality (see Table 6–4).

The QI approach assumes that most people want to perform well and will improve when the advantage is clearly shown. This is far more fair to all the stakeholders in the process than the retrospective QA practices of the past. Before-the-fact measures to provide accountability to the system constitute a sort of accounting control[12] that attempts to avoid suboptimal use of resources. The use of valid and reliable outcomes measurement tools, along with administrative controls, which use feedback to make adjustments and avoid mistakes in the future, has the potential to effect rapid changes in the quality of service delivery.

Table 6–4 The Effects of Good Quality

	Outcomes			
	Meets Customer Needs	*Customer Experiences*	*Benefits to Organization*	*Higher Quality Results in*
Features (*structure*)	Right features	Increased satisfaction	Higher income	Increased costs
Free from deficiences (*process*)	Without deficiencies	Reduced dissatisfaction	Lower costs	Lower costs

Source: Facilitating and Leading Quality Improvement Teams, © 1993, Juran Institute, Inc. Used with permission. All rights reserved.

Applying Juran's and Deming's concepts to health care has been a struggle, partly because of the socialization of physician leaders and partly because of the misincentives lingering in nominally nonprofit provider structures and profit-driven insurance systems. Also, as Richard Coffey and his team at the University of Michigan concluded from their experience of implementing QI, QI demands a paradigm shift, which is difficult for most people.[13] According to Joel Barker, a paradigm is a set of rules and regulations that defines boundaries and tells you what to do to be successful within those boundaries.[14] Those who have been successful in the old paradigms have diminished motivation and ability to change, and may therefore be unwilling or unable to adapt to the requirements of QI.

In QI theory as specifically applied to health care, *re-dos* would include additional treatment made necessary by inadequate or inappropriate care measures. Experienced QA physicians have set the cost of re-dos in hospitals at as much as 25 to 40%.[15] *The meeting of fitness-for-use specifications* would translate as the meeting of patient-defined needs. Together, the absence of re-dos and the meeting of fitness-for-use specifications constitute quality. According to the Health Outcomes Institute, quality in health care is achieved by "doing the right thing right," where "the right thing" is outcomes management and one does it "right" by process control.[16]

Whereas QA relies on provider-defined outcomes of care such as morbidity, mortality, and clinical endpoints, QI relies on user- or customer-defined outcomes such as patient satisfaction, cost of care, functional health, feeling of well-being, and health-related quality of life. Letting user-defined health outcomes tools direct the goals of the QI program provides a simplicity of mission to a QI effort.

Traditional QA tended to focus on statistical outliers, whether of cost or morbidity/mortality. It is guided by the 80/20 rule (or "Pareto Principle") that 80 percent of the costs is generated by 20 percent of the patients. QI focuses on continual improvement of all processes—even where no problem is identified. Such an approach can improve the quality of care of the majority of patients and decrease the outliers along the way (see Figure 6–1).

Table 6–5 compares QA and QI (specifically TQM) philosophy and methods. Table 6–6 compares QA and QI with other approaches by hospitals to cope with the current cost control environment.

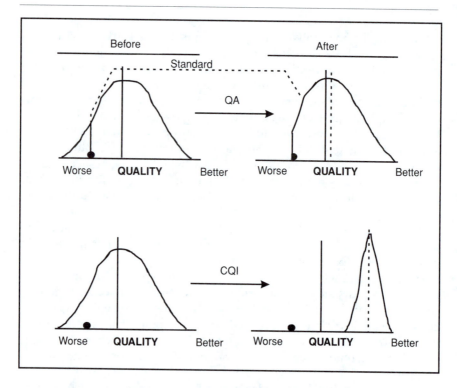

Figure 6–1 The Impact of Effective Standards Versus Continuous Quality Improvement on the Location and Spread of a Quality Indicator. *Source*: Reprinted from *Introduction to Outcomes*, p. 27, with permission of the Health Outcomes Institute, © 1994.

Table 6–5 Comparison of Traditional QA and TQM

Characteristic	Traditional Quality Assurance	Total Quality Management
Purpose	Improve quality of patient care for patients	Improve quality of all services and products for patients and other customers
Scope	Clinical processes and outcomes Actions directed toward people studied Mandated by JCAHO and others	All systems and processes—clinical and nonclinical Actions directed toward process improvement Optional, but in order to meet JCAHO performance measurement, some aspects of TQM needed
Leadership	Physician and clinical leaders: chief of clinical staff, QA committee	All clinical and nonclinical leaders
Aims	Problem solving Identify indivduals whose outcomes are outside specified thresholds—implies special causes	Continuous improvement, even if no "problem" identified Addresses both special and common causes—most attention toward common causes
Focus	Peer review vertically focused by department or clinical process—each department does its own QA Unacceptable few—education or elimination of those who do not meet standards Inspection Outcome-oriented	Horizontally focused to improve all processes and people that affect outcomes Improve performance of everyone, not just the unacceptable few Prevention and design to improve the processes—then inspection to monitor process Process- and outcome-oriented
Customers and Requirements	Customers are professionals and review organizations—patient is focus Measures and standards established by healthcare professionals only	Customers are patients, professionals, review organizations, and others—everyone No long-term fixed standards—continuously improving standards established by customers and professionals

continues

Table 6–5 continued

Characteristic	Traditional Quality Assurance	Total Quality Management
Methods	Chart audits Nominal group technique Hypothesis testing Indicator monitoring	Indicator monitoring and data use Brainstorming Nominal group technique Force field analysis Coaching/mentoring Flowcharting Checklist Histogram/Pareto chart Cause-effect, fishbone diagram Run/control chart Stratification Quality function deployment Hoshin planning
People Involved	QA program and appointed committees Actions decided by committees appointed for specific periods Limited involvement	Everyone involved with process Actions decided by team of people familiar with process—no time period specified Total institutional involvement
Outcomes	Includes measurement and monitoring May improve performance of the few individuals addressed Creates defensive posturing	Includes measurement and monitoring Improves performance of everyone involved in process Focus on process improvement—reduces threat to individuals, promotes team spirit, and can break down turf lines Includes QA efforts
Continuing Activities	Monitor for deviations from thresholds/standards Follow up when there are special cause deviations	Monitor processes for deviations (QA) and continually improve standards (QI) Follow up when there are special or common cause deviations

Source: Reprinted from *Total Quality in Healthcare* by R. Coffey and E. Gaucher, pp. 58–59, with permission of Jossey-Bass Inc., Publishers, © 1993.

Table 6-6 Types of Organizational Change in Health Care Organizations

	QA	QI	Automation	Reengineering	Reorganization	Downsizing
Focus	Satisfy licensure	Strategic	Reduce time	Strategic	Cuts costs	Cuts costs
Approach	Top-down	Top-down & bottom-up	Functional	Top-down	Top-down	Top-down
Goals	Reduce errors	Satisfy customers	Improve productivity	Improve productivity dramatically	Reduce costs	Reduce costs
Actions	Track outliers	Improve processes	Automate	Replace processes	Collapse layers	Reduce staffing
Type of change	Incremental	Incremental	Automation	Radical	Layoffs	Layoffs
Time line	Long	Long	1–3 years	2–4 years	Short	Short
Employee	Not invested	Participant in QI teams	Participant in information systems teams	Participant in reengineering teams	Victim	Victim
Automation	Variable	Considered	Yes	Key component	No	No

QI produces incremental change, which for some means change that occurs too slowly. Reengineering, now being touted as a way to improve processes rapidly relies on information systems to achieve this goal. This approach is advocated for large systems.[17] However, reengineering efforts that do not incorporate QI are set up for failure.

QI AND CASE MANAGEMENT

The QI approach has a significant conceptual fit with case management. Indeed, case managers engage in many of the behaviors of quality improvement: brainstorming; indicator monitoring; consensus building; use of checklists, activity logs, and flowcharts; coaching and mentoring; and return-on-investment projections.

The first task of a case manager is to select those patients who would most benefit from case management from a resource utilization point of view, and the second is to define and facilitate patient treatment goals.

Traditionally, case management triggers have been dollar threshold, diagnosis, and selected demographic and clinical risk factors. But these indices have been ineffective in controlling costs and improving outcome. Dollar thresholds are not very useful to trigger successful case management intervention because the treatment plan has already been set (and has probably failed) before the dollar trigger is reached. It is very difficult for a case manager to steer a case that has been mishandled once a variety of interventions have been tried and have failed. Moreover, significant practical and theoretical constraints prevent medically meaningful inferences about who is going to do well or poorly in the medical care system based on selected risk factors. Certainly, age is the most significant predictor of hospital death,[18] and "clinical stability" has been tracked by large database outcomes tools such as Medisgroups. But while age, physiologic health measures, DRGs, or prior resource utilization may be able to predict resource use for aggregate populations, they are not accurate predictors of resource use when applied to individual patients.[19] Comorbidities are a dimension of risk that extends beyond the medical model's ability to predict or control the risk for specific individuals. Predicting and controlling appropriateness of care and resource use is in its infancy, and many physicians and hospitals have disputed the inferences of this type of data.[20]

Patient-defined measures of functioning, feeling states and self-reported health (discussed in detail in the next section) are more useful for predicting resource utilization and indentifying patients who tend not to do well in the health system and therefore may benefit from case management. (These patients tend to be chronically ill medical patients rather than

Table 6–7 QI Outcomes Measures

Outcome Measure	Definition	Examples
Functional health status	patient's ability to perform self-care activities normal for age and role status	ability to carry a bag of groceries up a flight of stairs, walk 3 blocks without becoming short of breath or developing chest pain
Well-being	report of pain, self-rated vitality (energy/fatigue), social functioning, psychological distress	chronic pain, depression, sleep disorders, socially withdrawn, poor self-rated health
Patient satisfaction	access/convenience to care, waiting times, continuity of care, interpersonal style of caregiver, financial aspects, technical aspects	staff, physician friendliness, taking time to talk with patient, would patient recommend this doctor or facility to friend
Cost	actual costs of resource utilization rather than charges	relative efficiency of personnel, absence of mistakes, tests ordered appropriately

surgical patients whose treatment path is fairly straightforward.) Such measures are also useful for tracking quality prospectively. They can uncover patient-defined issues that help the case manager indentify appropriate treatment goals and realistic outcomes (Clinical endpoints are still important, but they must relate to the patient's ability to maintain his or her own expected level of well-being and of social and role functioning.) Health status instruments can also provide ongoing feedback so that participating providers (physicians and others) can learn how their interventions have affected the patient's functional health and well-being and modify the treatment plan to best suit the patient's needs.

QI process techniques such as seeking consensus from all parties, providing feedback to improve coordination of activity, and incorporating multidisciplinary planning and preventive measures into the treatment plan can enhance case managers' ability to reach treatment goals. In addition, QI team-building processes can be useful for case management programs, which ideally involve teamwork between the case manager and all the participants, and the operational and training support to ensure that team goals are met. Case management programs should be facilitated to go through the QI steps *forming* the group identity and goals, *brainstorming* problems and procedures, *norming* (i.e., setting norms and benchmarking standards), and *performing* the plan-do-collect-act cycle to eliminate variation in the care delivery process. Prospective outcomes measures help define the treatment task as much as the health history and physical exam. Practice guidelines are the road map.

QI OUTCOMES MEASURES

Outcomes measured by QI include functional health status, well-being, patient satisfaction, and cost. Table 6–7 summarizes and gives examples for these types of measures.

Functional Health Status Measures

Measurements of functional health have long been used in medical rehabilitation to justify the care rendered. These measurements have largely focused on evaluating the degree of assistance patients require to perform ADL (activity of daily living) skills.[21] The Expanded Disability Status Scale focuses on mobility,[22] the Level of Rehabilitation Scale (LORS) on communication,[23] and the Patient Evaluation Conference System (PECS) on interpersonal skills.[24] The last two scales focus more on the effectiveness of the rehabilitation program than on the patient.

The most widely used tool now available is the Functional Independence Measures (FIM) developed through grants from the National Institute on Disability and Rehabilitation Research (NIDRR). The Uniform Data System (UDS) for Medical Rehabilitation at the State University of New York in Buffalo now administers the FIM and the WeeFIM, which is used for children from six months to seven years of age.

The FIM and WeeFIM are a uniform data set that focuses on key functional attributes. Eighteen items are measured on a seven-point scale (Exhibits 6–2 and 6–3). The instrument has been validated and has gained wide acceptance among rehabilitation clinicians, administrators, and researchers. The tool is designed to be discipline-free and can be administered quickly and uniformly. UDS certifies agencies to administer it after training has been rendered, and provider facilities who are subscribers to the UDS transmit their data quarterly to UDS and receive reports on their results as compared to other facilities and in terms of patient diagnosis characteristics.[25] The facility can use the data to improve its internal processes and for marketing if desired.

The FIM and WeeFIM is based on the World Health Organization's definitions of *impairment, disability,* and *handicap* (see Exhibit 6–4). The FIM/WeeFIM recognize that impairments at the organ level do not necessarily lead to restrictions or lack of ability of the person to function normally (a disability). These tools weigh the level of disability and handicap which results from a given impairment. The result is so far the

Exhibit 6–2 Items Measured on FIM and WeeFIM

Functional Independence Measure (FIM)

MOTOR
  Self-Care
    A.   Eating   ❑
    B.   Grooming   ❑
    C.   Bathing   ❑
    D.   Dressing-Upper Body   ❑
    E.   Dressing-Lower Body   ❑
    F.   Toileting   ❑
  Sphincter Control
    G.   Bladder Management   ❑
    H.   Bowel Management   ❑
  Transfers
    I.   Chair, Wheelchair   ❑
    J.   Toilet   ❑
    K.   Tub, Shower   ❑

  Locomotion
    L.   Walk/Wheelchair/Crawl   ❑
    M.   Stairs   ❑
  { ○ Walk ○ Wheelchair ○ Crawl ○ Combination

COGNITIVE
  Communication
    N.   Comprehension   ❑ { ○ Auditory ○ Visual ○ Both

    O.   Expression   ❑ { ○ Vocal ○ Nonvocal ○ Both
  Social Cognition
    P.   Social Interaction   ❑
    Q.   Problem Solving   ❑
    R.   Memory   ❑

Source: From *Guide for the Uniform Data Set for Medical Rehabilitation for Children (WeeFIM* SM*),* *Version 4.0-Inpatient.* Buffalo, NY 14214: State University of New York at Buffalo, 1993. For more information contact: Uniform Data System, 232 Parker Hall, University at Buffalo-South Campus, 3435 Main Street, Buffalo, NY 14214-3007.

---

best way to measure the effectiveness of rehabilitation efforts in terms of burden of care and resource use. Etiologic diagnosis, other diagnoses, an impairment classification, and cost/resource use data are all collected to determine the effectiveness of the rehabilitation effort. The decision tree for the WeeFIM that asks the clinician to make a determination of severity of disability does so in terms of the burden of care, or substituted time and energy.

The FIM/WeeFIM has been helpful in measuring locomotion/mobility issues and ADLs, but its measurement of the communication and social

Exhibit 6–3 Instructions for the Use of the WeeFIM Decision Trees

The WeeFIM decision trees were originally designed to provide a structured interview format for use during the WeeFIM standardization process. The trees will be useful in any situation where clinicians are not able to directly observe the child's behavior, as in follow-up assessments by telephone.

Refer to the techniques to facilitate administration of the WeeFIM on page 6 and use the guidelines to determine the most appropriate place in the trees to begin the interviews. Follow the branches to obtain the correct ratings.

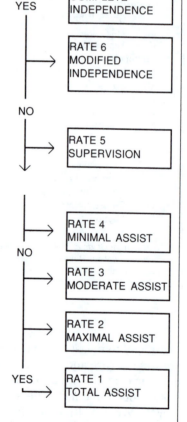

NO HELPER

Does the child complete the activity as described without any help or assistive devices, safely and in a reasonable amount of time?

YES → RATE 7 COMPLETE INDEPENDENCE

Does the child need more than a reasonable amount of time or an assistive device or is there a concern for safety?

→ RATE 6 MODIFIED INDEPENDENCE

HELPER   NO

Does the child need set up, supervision, cuing or coaxing, without physical contact, if motor activity or without significant prompting/direction, if cognitive activity?

→ RATE 5 SUPERVISION

Does the child complete most of the activity by him/herself with no more help than touching, if motor activity, or without significant prompting/direction, if cognitive activity?

→ RATE 4 MINIMAL ASSIST

NO

Does the child complete half or more of the activity by him/herself and require more help than touching?

→ RATE 3 MODERATE ASSIST

Does the child complete less than half of the activity by him/herself?

→ RATE 2 MAXIMAL ASSIST

Does the child complete little, or none, of the activity by him/herself?

YES → RATE 1 TOTAL ASSIST

Source: Copyright © 1993, Uniform Data System for Medical Rehabilitation, U.B. Foundation Activities, Inc.

Exhibit 6–4 World Health Organization Definitions

IMPAIRMENT
- Abnormalities or disturbances of structure or function. Disturbances at organ level, includes anatomical, physiological or psychological.

DISABILITY
- Any restriction or lack of ability to function normally as a consequence of impairment. Disturbances at the level of the person; concerned with restriction of compound integrated activities—tasks, skills and behaviors.

HANDICAP
- A disadvantage for a given individual resulting from an impairment or disability, limiting or preventing the individual from fulfilling a role that is normal for that individual.
- Handicap reflects the cultural, social or economic consequences of the impairment or disability. Handicap is shaped by values and attitudes.

Source: Adapted from *International Classification of Impairments, Disabilities and Handicaps*, p. 14, with permission of the World Health Organization, © 1980.

---

cognition domains is limited and may not give a true picture of functional ability for many patients. The Functional Assessment Measure (FAM) was developed for the brain- and spinal-cord-injured population to address this issue. The FAM adds 12 items (swallowing, car transfer, community access, reading, writing, speech intelligibility, emotional status, adjustment to limitations, employability, orientation, attention, and safety judgment) to the FIM. Like the FIM, it is scored on a seven-point scale indicating level of independence.[26]

The FIM and FAM are appropriate tools to use with patients who are not able to rate themselves (keeping in mind that our ideal outcome is rated by the customer, not the provider of services). A validated psychometric measure of functional health was also developed by the Medical Outcomes Study and is reflected in the Medical Outcomes Study Short Form 36 or SF-36 (see Exhibit 6–5).

Medical Outcomes Study Short Form 36 (SF-36)

The Medical Outcomes Study, which was based on the outcome categories in Donabedian's structure-process-outcomes model, was the first to explore specifically the effects of cost containment on patient outcomes.[27] Outcomes were defined in terms of functioning: ADLs, feeling states, and self-rated health. The SF-36 and its permutations are a set of psychometric variables that can predict resource utilization. Used properly, this tool can

Exhibit 6–5 Medical Outcomes Study Short Form 36 (SF-36)

SF-36™ HEALTH STATUS SURVEY (Acute)

INSTRUCTIONS: This survey asks for your views about your health now and during the past week. This information will help keep track of how you feel and how well you are able to do your usual activities.

Answer every question by marking the appropriate oval. If you are unsure about how to answer a question, please give the best answer you can.

Before beginning this questionnaire... Please pencil in your ID number in the squares to the right and then darken in the appropriate oval below each number.

If you don't know what ID number to use, ask the person who gave you this questionnaire.

Now begin with the questions below.

1. In general, would you say your health is:

1. ① Excellent
   ② Very good
   ③ Good
   ④ Fair
   ⑤ Poor

2. Compared to one week ago, how would you rate your health in general now?

2. ① Much better now than 1 week ago
   ② Somewhat better now than 1 week ago
   ③ About the same
   ④ Somewhat worse now than 1 week ago
   ⑤ Much worse now than 1 week ago

3. The following items are about activities you might do during a typical day. Does your health now limit you in these activities? If so, how much? (Mark one oval on each line.)
   a. *Vigorous activities,* such as running, lifting heavy objects, participating in strenuous sports
   b. *Moderate activities,* such as moving a table pushing a vacuum cleaner, bowling, or playing golf
   c. Lifting or carrying groceries
   d. Climbing *several* flights of stairs
   e. Climbing *one* flight of stairs

3.

	Yes, Limited A Lot	Yes, Limited A Little	No, Not Limited At All
a.	①	②	③
b.	①	②	③
c.	①	②	③
d.	①	②	③
e.	①	②	③

Exhibit 6–5 continued

f. Bending, kneeling, or stooping	f. ①. . . . . .②. . . . . .③
g. Walking *more than a mile*	g. ①. . . . . .②. . . . . .③
h. Walking *several blocks*	h. ①. . . . . .②. . . . . .③
i. Walking *one block*	i. ①. . . . . .②. . . . . .③
j. Bathing or dressing yourself	j. ①. . . . . .②. . . . . .③

4. During the past week, have you had any of the
following problems with your work or other regular
daily activities as a result of your physical
health? (Mark one oval on each line.)
   a. Cut down the *amount of time* you spent on
      work or other activities
   b. *Accomplished less* than you would like
   c. Were limited in the *kind* of work or other activities
   d. Had *difficulty* performing the work or other
      activities (for example, it took extra effort)

4.

        Yes   No

a. ①. . . . . .②
b. ①. . . . . .②
c. ①. . . . . .②

d. ①. . . . . .②

5. During the past week, have you had any of the
problems with your work or other regular daily
activities as a result of any emotional problems
(such as feeling depressed or anxious)? (Mark
one oval on each line.)
   a. Cut down the *amount of time* you spent on
      work or other activities
   b. *Accomplished less* than you would like
   c. Didn't do work or other activities as *carefully*
      as usual

5.

        Yes   No

a. ①. . . . . .②
b. ①. . . . . .②

c. ①. . . . . .②

6. During the past week, to what extent has your
physical health or emotional problems intefered
with your normal social activities with family,
friends, neighbors, or groups? (Mark one oval.)

6.
① Not at all   ④ Quite a bit
② Slightly   ⑤ Extremely
③ Moderately

7. How much bodily pain have you had during the
past week? (Mark one oval.)

7. ① None   ④ Moderate
② Very mild   ⑤ Severe
③ Mild   ⑥ Very severe

8. During the past week, how much did pain
interfere with your normal week (including both
work outside the home and housework)? (Mark
one oval.)

8. ① Not at all   ④ Quite a bit
② A little bit   ⑤ Extremely
③ Moderately

9. These questions are about how you feel and how
things have been with you during the past week.
For each question, please give the one answer
that comes closest to the way you have been
feeling. How much of the time during the past
week...(Mark one oval on each line.)
   a. Did you feel full of pep?
   b. Have you been a very nervous person?
   c. Have you felt so down in the dumps nothing
      could cheer you up?
   d. Have you felt calm and peaceful?
   e. Did you have a lot of energy?
   f. Have you felt downhearted and blue?
   g. Did you feel worn out?
   h. Have you been a happy person?
   i. Did you feel tired?

9.

	All of the Time	Most of the Time	A Good Bit of the Time	Some of the Time	A Little of the Time	None of the Time
a.	①	②	③	④	⑤	⑥
b.	①	②	③	④	⑤	⑥
c.	①	②	③	④	⑤	⑥
d.	①	②	③	④	⑤	⑥
e.	①	②	③	④	⑤	⑥
f.	①	②	③	④	⑤	⑥
g.	①	②	③	④	⑤	⑥
h.	①	②	③	④	⑤	⑥
i.	①	②	③	④	⑤	⑥

continues

Exhibit 6–5 continued

10. During the past week, how much of the time has your physical or emotional problems interfered with your social activities (like visiting with friends, relatives, etc.)? (Mark one oval.)	10. ① All of the time ④ A little of the time ② Most of the time ⑤ None of the time ③ Some of the time

11. Please choose the answer that best describes how true or false each of the following statements is for you. (Mark one oval on each line.)

11.

	Definitely True	Mostly True	Not Sure	Mostly False	Definitely False
a. I seem to get sick a little easier than other people.	a. ①	②	③	④	⑤
b. I am as healthy as anybody I know.	b. ①	②	③	④	⑤
c. I expect my health to get worse.	c. ①	②	③	④	⑤
d. My health is excellent.	d. ①	②	③	④	⑤

12a. Which are you?
b. How old were you on your last birthday?
	12.a. ○ Male ○ Female
	b. ○ Less than 35 ○ 65-74
	    ○ 35-44 ○ 75-84
	    ○ 45-54 ○ 85 and older
	    ○ 55-64

13. Have you ever filled out this form before?	13. ○ Yes
	      ○ No
	      ○ Don't remember

Thank you for your time.	14. DO NOT MARK HERE Ⓐ Ⓑ Ⓒ Ⓓ Ⓔ NOT LAST CARD ○

also discriminate stages and severity of disease and moderate-sized treatment effects.

The SF-36 is a prospective tool to track quality. The measures are performed parallel initially and longitudinally. Tarlov has stated that its widespread use as a strategic tool "could do more to improve the cost-effectiveness of health care than any other innovation."[28]

The instrument contains 36 items that measure eight health concepts (see Exhibit 6–6). It can be self-administered via phone or by mail within five minutes. The scoring sheet can be scanned so as to eliminate data input errors. It has been shown to be an effective indicator of health status (.7 to .8 positive correlation with actual health examinations) and is being used in ongoing longitudinal studies involving thousands of patients.[29]

The SF-36 has been adapted for use with older U.S. patients, patients in the United Kingdom, and patients of Mexican American background. It has also been normed for a number of comorbid conditions (hypertension, diabetes, acute myocardial infarction, back pain, etc.). It is available in baseline and acute versions.[30]

The HSQ and TyPE Specifications

The Health Status Questionnaire (HSQ) and Technology of Patient Experience (TyPE) survey tools were developed by Interstudy, now called

Exhibit 6–6   Health Concepts Measured by the SF-36

Health Concept	Questions Asked:
1. Physical functioning	Ability to climb stairs, walk distances, bending, lifting, stooping?
2. Role limitations due to physical health problems	Difficulty performing, took longer time, accomplished less than would like?
3. Social functioning	Social activities limited by health, visiting friends and relatives?
4. Bodily pain	Incidence or pain and how much it interferes with normal work?
5. General mental health	Nervous person, downhearted and blue, happy?
6. Role limitations due to emotional problems	Cut down on amount of time spent on activities, not as careful as usual, accomplished less than would like?
7. Vitality (energy/fatigue)	Full of pep, tired, worn out?
8. General health perceptions	Health perceptions compared with other people, change in health during past year?

Source: Adapted from *Measuring Function and Well-being*, A. Stewart and J. Ware, eds., p. 21, with permission of Duke University Press, © 1980.

the Health Outcomes Institute. The use of these tools and others is part of the OMS or Outcomes Management System being promoted by this non-profit organization. The mission of the Health Outcomes Institute is the widescale implementation of outcomes data using these clinical and psychometric tools. The HSQ is the SF-36 with three questions on depression added. The baseline survey also asks demographic questions (i.e., age, marital status, income, and some health risk inventory questions regarding cigarette smoking, seatbelt use, recent pap smear, etc.).

The TyPE specifications ask clinically related questions of the patient and sometimes the physician. Eighteen different diagnostic categories are now in use: angina, asthma, carpal tunnel, cataract, chronic sinusitis, COPD, depression, diabetes, hip fracture, hip replacement, hypertension/lipid disorder, low back pain, osteoarthritis of the knee, panic disorder, prostatism, rheumatoid arthritis, stroke, and substance abuse (alcohol).[31] These survey tools use SF-36 types of questions that directly correspond to functional and symptom-related issues. More TyPE categories are under development, and the ones in use undergo periodic adjustments. The American Group Practice Association uses similar versions of the TyPEs, and software vendors that assist in total program assessment also offer versions.[32]

A number of large-scale studies are now going on with managed-care systems and employer groups. Operational issues regarding the collection of data across the continuum of care, the utility of the data, and feedback methods to clinicians and managers are being field-tested.[33]

Current Issues Regarding Health Status Measures

For a number of historical and methodological reasons, health status measures have not yet reached wide acceptance. Doctors often disregard patient reports of distress, and aggregate data of such distress are seen as "too soft."[34] The "hard" data of numbers generated by such procedures as lab tests fit the training and socialization of physicians. Yet psychometric measures of health have been shown to be much more valid indicators of the real health of human beings than the biologic metric that we have used for so many years.

Up until recently, functional improvements in health status could not be measured in a disease-specific way. Some of the work with the TyPEs addresses this issue, but there needs to be a standardization of the instruments, the weighting schemes for scoring, and the interpretive meanings of the score differences as patients are assessed over time.

Technical and operational problems related to collection and input of the data captured by health status measures are being overcome as the price of software, scanners, and computer equipment moderates. But missing data remain a problem. An unreturned survey instrument often means that the patient is depressed or in poorer health.[35]

Patient-Defined Outcome Measures and Health-Related Quality of Life

By asking patients to rate their physical and functional status, their psychological well-being, and some social role functioning, the SF-36 and HSQ have begun to explore how quality of life relates to outcomes. They are easier to use and just as reliable as older and longer instruments such as the Sickness Impact Profile.[36] On both the HSQ and the SF-36 (see Exhibit 6–5), many more questions relate to the absence of negative factors (e.g., pain, difficulty, limitation) than to the presence of positive factors. This points up the problem of using health status scales to get at quality-of-life issues: one cannot infer from them the causal sequence that leads patients to make certain evaluations in their lives. Case managers need to follow up on below-threshold scores to find out what caused a patient to rate his or her health and well-being poorly.

Hyland postulated that health-related quality of life (HRQOL) is determined both by morbidity and by psychological factors such as traits, mood, coping style, and cognitive style.[37] It is also judged on the basis of current circumstances: for example, renal failure patients who have undergone transplants, hemodialysis, and peritoneal dialysis are more likely to rate themselves "very happy" than the general population. Quality of life, then, is a function of personality, expectations, and the impact of disease states on everyday life.

NOTES

1. M.J. Mehlman, Assuring the Quality of Medical Care: The Impact of Outcome Measurement and Practice Standards, *Law, Medicine and Health Care* 18 (1990):370.

2. A. Donabedian, Evaluating the Quality of Care, *Milbank Memorial Fund Quarterly* 44, part 2 (1966):166–203.

3. Institute of Medicine, *Controlling Costs and Changing Patient Care: The Role of Utilization Management* (Washington, D.C.:1989), 4.

4. J.C. Linder, Outcomes Measurement: Compliance Tool or Strategic Initiative? *Health Care Management Review* 16, no. 4 (1991):23.

5. L.I. Iezzoni, Risk and Outcomes, in *Risk Adjustment for Measuring Health Care Outcomes*, ed. L.I. Iezzoni (Ann Arbor, Mich.: Health Administration Press, 1994), 7.

6. N. Goldfield et al., *Measuring and Managing Health Care Quality* (Gaithersburg, Md.: Aspen Publishers, Inc., 1993), 1–2; L.I. Iezzoni, A Tabular Summary of Severity Systems, cited in Goldfield, *Measuring and Managing Health Care Quality*, Appendix C, 1–3.

7. E. Guadagnoli and B.J. McNeil, Outcomes Research: Hope for the Future or the Latest Rage? *Inquiry* 31 (1994):14–24.

8. R.A. Deyo and D.L. Patrick, Barriers to the Use of Health Status Measures in Clinical Investigation, Patient Care, and Policy Research, *Medical Care* 27 (1989):S254–S268.

9. L. Koran, The Reliability of Clinical Methods, Data and Judgments (Part 2), *New England Journal of Medicine*, 293 (1975):695–701.

10. Joint Commission on Accreditation of Healthcare Organizations, *Accreditation Manual for Hospitals* (Oakbrook Terrace, Ill.:1992).

11. J.M. Juran and F.M. Gyrna, *Juran's Quality Control Handbook*, 4th ed. (New York: McGraw-Hill Publishing Co., 1988), 2–8.

12. S.A. Finkler, *Cost Accounting for Health Care Organizations* (Gaithersburg, Md.: Aspen Publishers, Inc., 1994), 406.

13. R.J. Coffey and E.J. Gaucher, *Total Quality in Healthcare* (San Francisco: Jossey-Bass Inc., Publishers, 1983), 37ff.

14. Coffey and Gaucher, *Total Quality in Healthcare*, 58–61.

15. D. Nash, Involving Physicians in TQM: Can It Be Done? (Paper presented at the meeting of the Greater Philadelphia Health Assembly, Philadelphia, October, 1992); also, Michael Cohen, M.D., Director of Quality Assurance at the Philadelphia Veterans Hospital, personal communication with author, 1992.

16. Health Outcomes Institute, *Introduction to Outcomes* (Bloomington, Minn.:1994).

17. M. Kennedy, Reengineering in Healthcare, *Quality Letter for Healthcare Leaders* 6, no. 7 (1994):2–10.

18. L.I. Iezzoni, Dimensions of Risk, in L.I. Iezzoni, ed., *Risk Adjustment*, 30.

19. J.P. Newhouse et. al., Adjusting Capitation Rates Using Objective Health Measures and Prior Utilization, *Health Care Financing Review* 10, no.3 (1989):41–53; J.E. Ware, Conceptualizing and Measuring Generic Health Outcomes, *Cancer* 67, suppl. (1991):774–779.

20. L.I. Iezzoni and L.G. Greenberg, Risk Adjustment and Current Health Policy Debates, in L.I. Iezzoni, ed., *Risk Adjustment*, 378–383.

21. K. Wagner, Outcome Analysis in Comprehensive Medical Rehabilitation, in *Rehabilitation Outcomes: Analysis and Measurement*, ed. M. Fuhrer (Baltimore: Brooks, 1989), 22.

22. J.F. Kurtske, Rating Neurological Impairment in Multiple Sclerosis: An Expanded Disablity Status Scale, *Neurology* 33 (1983):1444–1452.

23. R.G. Carey and E.J. Posavac, Program Evaluation of a Physical Medicine and Rehabilitation Unit: A New Approach, *Archives of Physical Medicine and Rehabilitation* 59 (1978):330–337.

24. R.F. Harvey and H.M. Jellinek, Functional Performance Assessment: A Program Approach, *Archives of Physical Medicine and Rehabilitation* 62 (1981):456–461.

25. State University at Buffalo, *Guide to the Uniform Data Set for Medical Rehabilitation for Children (WeeFIM^SM)*, Version 4.0 (Buffalo, N.Y.:SUNY, 1994), 1.1.

26. K.M. Hall et al., *The Functional Assessment Measure* (San Jose, Calif.: Santa Clara Valley Medical Center, 1993).

27. A.R. Tarlov et al., The Medical Outcomes Study: An Application of Methods for Monitoring the Results of Medical Care, *Journal of the American Medical Association* 262 (1989):foreword, 925–930; J.E. Ware, Jr., Measures for a New Era of Health Assessment, in *Measuring Functioning and Well-Being*, ed. A. Stewart and J.E. Ware (Durham, N.C.: Duke University Press, 1992), 9.

28. A. Tarlov, foreword to Stewart and Ware, *Measuring Function and Well-Being*, xv–xvi.

29. A. Stewart et al., The MOS Short-Form Health Survey: Reliability and Validity in a Patient Population, *Medical Care* 26 (1988):724–735.

30. J.E. Ware et al., *SF-36 Health Survey Manual and Interpretation Guide* (Boston: Health Institute, New England Medical Center, 1993).

31. Health Outcomes Institute. *An Introduction to the Health Outcomes Institute's Outcomes Management System.* Bloomington, Minn.: Health Outcomes Institute, 1993.

32 Velocity Software, Minnetonka, Minn., and Response Technologies, East Greenwich, R.I.

33. Health Outcomes Institute, Managed Health Care Association's Outcomes Project Expands into Next Phase, *Update* (Summer 1994):3.

34. Deyo and Patrick, Barriers.

35. A. Stewart et al., Summary and Discussion of MOS Measures, in Stewart and Ware, *Measuring Function and Well-Being*, 371.

36. J.N. Katz et al., Comparative Measurement Sensitivity of Short and Longer Health Status Instruments, *Medical Care* 30 (1992):917–925.

37. M.E. Hyland, A Reformulation of Quality of Life for Medical Science, *Quality of Life Research* 1 (1992):276–272.

7

Critical Paths and
Care Management

The term *critical path*, from industrial quality improvement theory, means an agreed-upon course of operational activities. In the health field it means an agreed-upon course of operational activities determined in response to patients' needs and circumstances, and it is used interchangeably with the term *clinical path*. A clinical path is an *algorithm*, or a procedure for performing a complicated operation by a precisely determined sequence of simpler steps. Algorithms are set up to exclude all personal or individual judgments. A patient assigned to a clinical path is expected to meet certain preset goals regarding his or her medical status or ability to perform certain functions at a specified point in time.

PLANNING THE CRITICAL PATH

As in any quality improvement project, the design of critical paths begins with a strategic planning process. Who are our stakeholders, which ones are most important to our mission, on what criteria do they judge us, and how well are we fulfilling their criteria? These questions anchor the process to customer-defined needs and enable planners to set outcome goals for system change.

Setting Outcome Goals

Outcome goals depend on such factors as the practice setting, the nature of the service, and the expectations of the payers and patients. Within an institution that is under capitation or a global (all-encompassing) budget, examples of goals might be, for a given service,

- to reduce the length of stay by 25 percent
- to reduce costs by 25 percent
- to reduce paperwork/documentation time by nurses by 30 percent
- to improve quality as measured by patient/family satisfaction.

Critical paths should be built around the types of cases that are most often seen or that have unacceptable rates of complications or variance from the expectations of customers.

Process Flow Analysis

After the goals have been set, the current critical path is analyzed. The first step is to determine who is performing the service and to represent everyone involved in the process on the planning team, since the adequacy of the new design will depend on the completeness of the information provided on the current state of operations. Then the team performs a process flow analysis: it identifies the critical elements or steps of the service, what drives people to perform the service well, what persons or practices inhibit performance, what supports (materials, training, computers, etc.) are necessary for doing the job without any re-dos that would divert energy and resources, and what indicators are used at what point in the process ("milestones") to confirm that the service is being carried out as expected.

Reformulation of the Critical Path

Once the current critical path is adequately understood, it can be reformulated to meet the outcome goals. First, the team ranks problem statements related to specific processes. Then it researches best practices "benchmarks" of other provider organizations and addresses suggested solutions to the problems that are ranked as highest priority. Next, the team works toward consensus to implement new processes and develops the new algorithm for these processes. It determines how desired outcomes will be measured and determines the milestones, for each state of the path, at which the functioning of the new system will be monitored. Benchmarking of other organizations' performance indicators can be useful in keeping performance expectations realistic.

The formulated path should be coherent to all the treatment team members, as well as to others who may be involved in the process or outcome of care. (For this reason, CareMAPs, or critical paths that use nursing diagnoses as part of the problem statements, may not work well for many settings.)

Once milestones and indicators are set, the team develops data collection and documentation processes, assigns a case manager, and implements the path. It analyzes the results and continues to review and revise the path as needed in a process of continuing feedback correction.

DIFFERENTIATING CARE MANAGEMENT FROM CASE MANAGEMENT

The determination of critical paths is a type of *care management*. Care management is independent of case management and has a different focus: its clinical algorithms are diagnosis-specific rather than patient-specific, its practice takes place within a specific setting rather than across the continuum of care, and it is designed to promote a quality outcome for all patients, whereas case management focuses on those who are or would tend to be outliers. Exhibit 7–1 presents a comparison of the features of care and case management.

Care management is an *iterative* (i.e., repetitive) process. It subjects all patients within a certain diagnostic classification to the same sequence of care activities and demands that patients be placed in a category even though there may not be a good "fit." It assumes, in fact, that all patients uniformly fit their classification, even though real-life situations can only approximate this orderly arrangement. In an iterative process, each iteration yields new data on the workings of the system, so feedback (or variance and outcomes measures) can continually drive the process to improve.

Case management, in contrast, is a heuristic process. Each patient is encountered as an individual, and although the outcome may not be entirely known or envisioned at the beginning of the process, goals and action steps are formulated on a step-by-step basis as information is gathered and the treatment process proceeds. Thus, a heuristic process, like an iterative process, relies on feedback, but the feedback can modify

Exhibit 7–1 Comparing Care and Case Management

Care Management	Case Management
Iterative process	Heuristic process
Within specific settings	Across continuum
Focused on diagnosis/process	Focused on patient/family
All patients eligible	Select probable outliers
Clinician driven	Assists physicians
System reengineering	Individual accountability
Biometric measures of outcomes	Psychometric measures of outcomes
Relies on information system and finance support	Relies on information system and finance support

the care plan at any point during treatment to match the patient-defined needs and goals and respond to the patient's unique circumstances.

Care management requires system adaptation or reengineering on the part of the provider organization in order to gather data and track patients in as near to "real time" as possible. Thus, it assumes a computer system to which multiple team members can contribute information and from which they can access information. Such computer support allows the case manager and the clinicians to track progress and intermediate clinical data points and to notify payer sources on a timely basis as to the status of patients for utilization management purposes.

Case management deals with the individual case. But it too requires support from information systems, to which a variety of administrators, including financial managers, may contribute, so that the efficiency of the treatment can be tracked.

Care management is focused on the care *process*. Treatment teams work out the most efficient and effective pathways for each diagnosis. But some patients and families are unable to stay on track with the time line and clinical goals of the treatment. They need case management, which provides a means of focusing on the patient rather than the process. Case management can assist physicians and other clinicians with communication, problem solving, special needs, and making the treatment team's time and effort more efficient and hassle-free.

Care management focuses on biometric, or biological, measures of treatment outcomes. These outcomes are defined by the provider rather than the customer and thus may have little relationship to the patient's functional health or perception of well being. They are merely good signposts or landmarks that cue the treatment team to the patient's progress. Case managers, however, should focus on psychometric measures of treatment outcomes, and deal with the complex psychosocial issues that tend to impede progress or compliance with the treatment plan.

SUMMARY

Case management focuses on actual or potential outlier patients, whereas care management focuses on categories of patients that have complex treatment needs or are frequently seen by the provider organization. Both approaches need to involve evidence-based interventions over experience-based interventions. The evidence that can drive planning and improvement of processes can come from expert panels or can be benchmarked from other provider performance clinical literature; it must also arise from data collected as patients are guided through the treatment plan. This evidence can markedly improve patient-defined outcomes, payer-defined outcomes, and clinician needs for the sense of satisfaction that arises from being part of a well-functioning treatment team.

8

An Ethical Framework for Case Management Practice

The "reform" movement in medical care that is evolving, with or without government's willingness or ability to define it, is essentially an effort at insurance reform. The cost and access inequities under the fee-for-service system have led to severe strains in the system in terms of cost shifting, medical inflation, and the financial viability of many medical providers.[1] This has in turn led to the movement for insurance reform and to ethical dilemmas. Poor access to care undermines the ethical behavior of health providers because they find themselves looking for ways to deny care that cannot be somehow paid for. Finance and cost reform have been proposed in order to solve the access problem.[2]

Most discussions regarding ethical problems faced by case managers have to do with sorting out rights and access issues in any given case. Indeed, right to services in a time of diminishing resources is particularly troubling. The case manager is often contractually expected to adminster access to services within the terms of the policy of the third-party payer, whereas the medical model that traditionally has governed ethical behavior for case managers expects providers to do good for their patients, not to be bound by resource-use considerations.[3]

Undoubtedly there is incongruity between the advocacy behavior that is part of the socialization of most nurses and other caregivers and the requirements of an insurance model cost containment enterprise. However, the level of conflict any given case manager feels on any given day has more to do with the specific practice setting and the goals of the organization than the inherent conflict of interest. For example, a telephone utilization review nurse who is trained and incentivized to deny coverage experiences more role conflict than an insurance case manager whose patients have been prequalified for coverage. The ethical conflicts of an internal case manager in a quality-driven provider organization would be fewer still.

The case manager is most often seen as both a patient advocate and a gatekeeper[4] and is charged to promote autonomy, beneficence, and justice.[5] The many ambiguous areas in which case managers are asked to practice and the failure of the medical model to address these issues present ongoing ethical problems for currently practicing case managers. Thus, practitioners would do well to develop some consensus about what a reasonable case manager would do when confronted with various ethical dilemmas. Case managers need to "bring to their work a well-developed sense of personal ethics."[6] Because of the complexity of most situations involving patients who require case management, each case manager should be grounded in a value system that goes beyond the traditional "justice" perspective of most discussions of ethical decision making.

ETHICAL PROBLEMS

Appropriateness of Care

A major ethical problem for case managers is that the acute care system, which relies on the biomedical model discussed in Chapter 1, does not work very well for most people—that is, the treatments it provides are often inappropriate and ineffective. The moral dissonance that case managers feel most often may stem from dealing with medical treatment plans that are poorly conceived and executed.

Physicians often respond to chronic problems by carrying out single interventions that do not take into account the patient's articulated needs and are not well coordinated. Although knowledge, skills acquisition, and social support can enable patients to adapt to chronic disease and can offset some of the impairments that it imposes, physicians have largely abrogated any duty to help patients in these areas, or in general to instruct and follow through to make sure their treatment plans are working. Nurses and other formal and informal caretakers often fill the gap. When the patient is not included or is not engaged in the treatment plan, the result is usually unsatisfactory. Noncompliance, miscommunications regarding expected outcomes, and inappropriate care result. Lawsuits are more likely. In any case, interventions designed to address acute problems usually do not work very well with chronic problems.

Another factor encouraging inappropriate care (and driving the increase in resource use of medical interventions) is the medicalization of daily life which has brought unrealistic expectations of cure for untreatable infirmities and unavoidable ailments.[7] Often the patient, family, and doctor believe that the patient has a certain "right" to a treatment that may have little chance of success. Is it moral to acquiesce to the provision of treatments or practices that have not yet been shown to be effective or safe? Some ethical observers think not.[8]

Truth Telling

Medicine's reliance on Hippocrates' dictum of *primam non nocere* ("above all, do no harm")[9] has created a tradition of truth evasions, beginning in a time when doctors could do little for patients other than predict the terminal course of a given disease. Because a terminal diagnosis, for example, could weaken the patient's will to live and thus be seen as a pronouncement of a death sentence, doctors felt justified in withholding this information. Thus Thomas Percival's 1803 discourse on medical ethics, though maintaining that patients had the right to hear the truth from their doctor, also insisted that the duty of truth telling could be suspended if the truth might seem to be an agent of harm. It was the place of doctors to offer hope when the prognosis of many diseases they saw was hopeless.[10] Eighty years later, Ganos commented on this ethical framework when he asserted that "medicine's heavy reliance on Hippocrates makes it susceptible to deceptive practices."[11]

Today, the paternalism inherent in therapeutic lying is giving way to a more modern attitude: that patients have equal moral standing in those issues that have to do with their bodies and their lives.[12] But as Marcia Liepman has pointed out, the doctor's own needs—convenience, money, fame, research goals, and simple self-protection—can still get in the way of honesty.[13]

Policies requiring the patient's informed consent to procedures might be seen as enforcing practitioners' truth telling, but they have not ensured it,[14] since it is so easy to manipulate consent by how information is divulged. And the deception can go much further: as Liepman remarks, "Deception is acting as if we *know* what is best for the patient, when in fact we *do not* know."[15]

Such truth evasions by practitioners have left the patient to cope alone with what Susan Sontag called "the night side of life . . . in the kingdom of the sick."[16] Sontag's famous discussion of the mythologies of disease and the devastation they invoke on the human spirit cries out for truth telling:

> All this lying to and by cancer patients is a measure of how much harder it has become in advanced industrial societies to come to terms with death. As death is now an offensively meaningless event, so disease is widely considered a synonym for death and is experienced as something to hide.[17]

As Sontag's statement illustrates, truth evasion is intimately bound up with denial of the patient's agency. Ivan Illich condemned the health care systems of the modern industrial state for what he called social and cultural iatrogenesis because "they destroy the potential of people to deal with their human weakness, vulnerability and uniqueness in a personal and autonomous way."[18] Illich's central thesis is that the system itself steals the meaning of the illness events by isolating the sick person away from home in the industrialized environment of a hospital. When the system is institution centered rather than patient centered, the goals of the system are incongruent with the patient's goals. Consequently, those activities and supports that gave meaning to the patient's everyday life are withdrawn. "Medical procedures turn into *black magic* when, instead of mobilizing his self-healing powers, they transform the sick man into a limp and mystified voyeur of his own treatment."[19] Withholding of information deepens patients' mystification and keeps them passive and dependent.

THE PROBLEM OF JUSTICE

The moral crisis in health care appears to reflect a philosophical tension within the system. Is health care a product or a service? Is it a right or a privilege? Are providers of care and insurance companies for-profit businesses or community service organizations? In the "libertarian" view, access to care is part of a society's reward system, and is an earned privilege. In the "egalitarian" view, access to care is every citizen's right.[20]

It is generally acknowledged that the justice ethic is a basic structural standard of this society, guiding legal, political, economic, and social institutions.[21] Reflecting Western society's fundamental espousal of the rights of the individual, this ethic rationally balances competing claims and judges what people owe or are owed according to principles of fairness, reciprocity, and equal treatment. Lawrence Kohlberg's model of moral development exemplifies this perspective in that it progresses from an egocentric understanding of fairness based on individual need, to a conception of fairness as determined by societal conventions, and finally to a conception of fairness based on consciously held principles of equality and reciprocity (Exhibit 8–1).[22]

Operationally, this perspective has problems. It leaves the individual acutely alone in the world, in search of his or her equal and justly apportioned share of resources. In a world of scarce resouces, some people can get what they need, and others cannot. Resource restriction leads to violence and litigation in which all parties are set against each other in a contest of rights.

Further, in health care, the satisfaction of claims to resources does not necessarily promote well-being. In fact, although objective measures of health have risen over the last 50 years, subjective measures of health have markedly declined.[23] As Carol Gilligan pointed out in her critique of Kohlberg's model, "the absolutes of truth and fairness, defined by the concepts of equality and reciprocity, are called into question by experiences that demonstrate the existence of differences between other and self. Then the awareness of multiple truths leads to a relativizing of equality in the direction of equity and gives rise to an ethic of generosity and care."[24] This ethic, as proposed by Gilligan, is responsive to individual differences in a way that is particularly congruent with the case manager role.

THE SOLUTION OF CARING

Gilligan challenged Kohlberg's dominant model by stating that moral development can move along a different continuum, that of caring. Citing empirical studies of women's moral development, she posited that women articulate their moral judgments in "a different voice": "The ideal of care is . . . an activity of relationship, of seeing and responding to need, taking care of the world by sustaining the web of connection, so that no one is left alone."[25] Gilligan contrasts this ethic with that of justice by stating that

Exhibit 8–1 Kohlberg's Six Stages of Moral Development

Stage 1:	Preconventional: Deference to authority
Stage 2:	Satisfying own needs and needs of others
Stage 3:	Conventional: Seeking approval from others by conforming to stereotypical roles
Stage 4:	Dutiful conduct to society, appreciation of value of maintaining the social order
Stage 5:	Association of morality with rights and standards endorsed by society as a whole
Stage 6:	Progress to self-chosen but universal principles of justice

"while the ethic of justice proceeds from the premise of equality—that everyone should be treated the same—an ethic of care rests on the premise of nonviolence—that no one should be hurt."[26]

The justice ethic applies abstract principles to resolve ethical dilemmas—for example, principles that assign more importance to some kinds of claims than others. But women, according to Gilligan, are reluctant to apply this ethic because they have difficulty becoming detached and depersonalizing situations. They are more likely to resolve ethical dilemmas in unique ways that consider the needs of all parties. This caring approach "is grounded in the assumption that self and other are interdependent."[27] Exhibit 8–2 summarizes differences between the justice and caring approaches.

Whether the ethic of caring is or is not gender based, an examination of the key words in Exhibit 8–2 reveals that the caring approach best represents the way most nurses interact with their patients.

Gilligan's caring framework does have precedent in the literature of moral philosophy. One such precedent is a book called *I and Thou* by the religious existentialist philosopher Martin Buber.[28] It describes two basic kinds of relationships: *I–Thou* and *I–It* relationships.

In *I–It* relationships, we depersonalize people, or relate to them as things. Objectifying and making judgments on people are aspects of this depersonalization. In this worldview, the *It* is always seen in terms of the *I's* preconceived notion of the universe. There is never a present with the *It*; only a past exists, because objective knowledge exists only in the past.

There is never a genuine relationship betwen the *I* and the *It*. The *I* is not engaged with the other; he or she is only a spectator. There can never be a full encountering of the other person if we bring our preconceived judgments to the relationship with another person. We will always feel our aloneness in the world.

In an *I–Thou* relationship, the other is engaged as a participant in relationship with the *I* in the present. The whole being is involved in the relationship, and there is no withholding of the self. The universe is thus

Exhibit 8–2 Justice Ethic Versus Caring Ethic

Justice	Caring
(Male)	(Female)
Thinking	Feeling
Egoism	Altruism
Theoretical reasoning	Practical reasoning
Grounds for agreement	Grounds for understanding
Rights/respect	Listening and speaking, hearing and being heard

seen in relationship with the *I*. There is no screening of communication with the other based on preconceived notions. Buber maintained that life is an endless transition, or path of learning, from an *I–It* to an *I–Thou* perspective.

There is clearly strong coherence between the moral theory of connectedness that Gilligan offered and Buber's *I–Thou* encounter. What this means for women and for case managers is that the caring perspective is at least as valid, sophisticated, and moral an ethical construct as the justice perspective.

ETHICAL CASE MANAGEMENT

Most of the nursing literature provides little guidance for case managers who are dealing with ethical issues. This is perhaps because nursing was originally practiced in a military context, and its metaphors have emphasized duty, loyalty, and blind obedience to authority.[29] Further, the primary practice site of nursing (hospitals) has not permitted nurses to have the autonomy of practice to act as moral agents.[30] But the advocacy role of nursing, which is fairly new on the scene, encourages patients to exercise self-determination. So does the shared-risk environment that is emerging in managed care (although here the encouragement of self-determination is in some conflict with the case manager's role of resource coordinator and gatekeeper). And patient self-determination demands honest communication between the case manager and the patient/family.

Honesty in the Case Manager–Patient Relationship

Honesty is an intentional act. It is more than freedom from fraud or deception; it is freedom from pretense, ornamentation, or disguise. It is the foundation for any caring behavior because it communicates respect and acknowledges the autonomy of the other.

Honesty involves listening. It involves being sensitive to different levels and styles of a patient's communication. Honesty demands patience, courage, and moral and intellectual integrity. Ethical behavior by case managers requires that they engage the patient in a dialogue of sustained conversation in which a care plan is mutually *discovered*. Ethical analysis and decision making involve insight, "seeing" the patient's point of view so that there is an adequate "fit" between the patient's aspirations and the plan of care.[31] Since case managers are usually not chosen by the patient (and may be seen as adversaries), such honesty demands tact and sensitivity.

Patients have their own story to tell about the meaning of their illness event, and are watchful when telling it to see if it is being listened to. The interview and subsequent interactions between patient and case manager are the opportunity to build a rapport so that honest negotiation and development of a plan of care can take place.

People are eager to retell the story of their illness because they are seeking affirmation and further clarification of the meanings they have given it. It is very helpful for case managers to speak directly to the stated and unstated *meaning* of the patient's story in order to build the relationship and guide a plan of care that is congruent with the patient's intentions.

Promoting Patient Self-Responsibility

The use of a caring over a justice perspective when engaging patients in the process of caring for themselves and coping with (usually incurable) illness has some strategic implications. Arthur S. Levine has pointed out that many people have the tendency to divest themselves of portions of their individual autonomy by projecting it upon the doctor or other caregiver. The heroic myths of hospital cures and larger-than-life performances by caregivers give brief comfort to those people who are uncomfortable accepting responsibility for their own lives and wish that their doctor or nurse would accept the responsibility instead. But caregivers are bound to fail in this larger-than-life role. The almost supernatural authority conferred on them leads to scapegoating by the patient and family whenever the outcome of treatment does not live up to the patient's often unspoken but nonetheless inflated expectations.[32]

The result of this subtle contract that makes the caregiver the hero and the patient passive is distorted. Real issues that are relevant to setting appropriate treatment goals are shunted aside. Illusions of self-enhancement dissolve in the face of chronic incapacitating conditions that have no cure.

Case managers can promote self-responsibility and avoid miscommunication and unrealistic expectations of patients and families by engaging the patient in truth telling and seeking the patient-defined meaning of illness. Techniques to increase patient and family participation (discussed later in this book) must have a demonstrated framework of caring evident to the patient in order to work. That is, the patient and family must believe that the case manager is honest and proceeding ethically.

The Case Manager–Physician Relationship

The role that case managers assume with physicians differs with practice settings and types of insurance. Case managers are sometimes seen as a threat, especially if the treatment plan has not been working or is otherwise inappropriate (as is too often the case in workers' compensation and auto accident cases). They can be welcomed (for example, by trauma surgeons) or vilified (especially if they are telephonic UR case managers).

Most physician–case manager conflicts are set up by differences in perspective: between justice and caring, or between the need for agreement and the need for understanding. Case managers should approach doctors carefully in order to smooth the way for collaboration. The emerging model of capitated payments provides incentives to restrict patients' resouce use. Case managers, by taking on the role of truth teller and setting a caring tone, put discussions relating to treatment plans for chronic patients at a different level. Faced with increasing levels of disability no matter what the treatment, a patient may opt to use fewer medical resources than current medical practice would suggest. The result is less pressure on the doctor to perform unlikely cures and less resource utilization. This will make the doctor look good.

Case managers who know what motivates their patients can reach for optimal quality-of-life outcomes that may not involve high-cost medical interventions. If the optimal result is patient-defined health status, the case manager is the right person with the right training at the right place to give optimal support to listening, collaborating, networking, teaching, and coaching activities. The "transformational leadership" activities that enable case managers to do this are discussed in Chapter 10.

NOTES

1. D.C. Coddington et al., *The Crisis in Healthcare* (San Francisco: Jossey-Bass Inc., Publishers, 1990).
2. T.A. Brennan, An Ethical Perspective on Health Care Insurance Reform, *American Journal of Law and Medicine* 19 (1993):39–74.
3. Brennan, An Ethical Perspective, 41; J. Banja, Whose Side Are You On? The Case Manager's Dilemma of Serving Two Masters (Interview), *Inside Case Management* 1, no. 4 (1994):6.
4. R.A. Kane and C.K. Thomas, What Is Case Management and Why Does It Raise Ethical Issues, in *Ethical Conflicts in the Management of Home Care*, ed. R.A. Kane and A.L. Caplan (New York: Springer Publishing Co., Inc., 1993), 3–6.
5. V. Tillman, Ethics, in *Case Management for Healthcare Professionals*, ed., R. Howe (Chicago: Precept Press, 1994), 35–38; Kane and Thomas, What Is Case Management, 5.
6. W.G. Bartholome, A Revolution in Understanding: How Ethics Has Transformed the Health Care Decision Process, *Qualtiy Review Bulletin* (Jan. 1992):6–11.
7. A.J. Barsky, The Paradox of Health, *New England Journal of Medicine* 318 (1988):414–418.
8. R.L. Levine, An Ethical Perspective, in *Quality of Life Assessments in Clinical Trials*, ed. B. Spilker (New York: Raven Press, 1990), 153–161.
9. Hippocrates, Selections from the Hippocratic Corpus, in *Ethics in Medicine: Historical Perspectives and Contemporary Concerns*, ed. S.J. Reiser et al. (Cambridge, Mass.: MIT Press, 1977), 5–7.

10. T. Percival, A Physician Should Be the Minister of Hope and Comfort to the Sick, in *Ethics in Medicine*, Reiser et al., 203–205.

11. D. Ganos, Introduction: Deception in a Teaching Hospital, in *Progress in Clincal and Biological Research: Proceedings of the Eighth and Ninth Conferences on Ethics, Humanism and Medicine, Held at the University of Michigan, 1981–82*, ed. D. Ganos (New York: Alan Liss, Inc., 1983), 77–80.

12. Bartholome, Revolution in Understanding, 9.

13. M. Liepman, Deception in a Teaching Hospital: Where We Are and Where We Are Going, in Ganos, *Progress*, 87–94.

14. H. Brody, Transparency: Informed Consent in Primary Care, *Hastings Center Report* (Sept.–Oct. 1989):87–94.

15. Liepman, Deception, 89.

16. S. Sontag, *Illness as Metaphor* (New York: Farrar, Straus & Giroux, 1978).

17. Sontag, *Illness as Metaphor*, 8.

18. I. Illich, *Medical Nemesis: The Expropriation of Health* (New York: Pantheon Books, 1978), 33. *Iatrogenesis* means "physician origin." Iatrogenic illness is usually considered to be a detrimental effect of medical or hospital practice; drug reactions, nosocomial infections, medical malpractice, and surgical misadventures are examples.

19. Illich, *Medical Nemesis*, 114.

20. A. Williams, Priority Setting in Public and Private Health Care: A Guide through the Ideological Jungle, *Journal of Health Economics* 7 (1988):173–183.

21. A. Buchanan, Justice: A Philosophical Review, in *Cross Cultural Perspectives in Medical Ethics: Readings*, 284.

22. L. Kohlberg, *The Philosophy of Moral Development* (San Francisco: Harper & Row, 1981).

23. Barsky, Paradox of Health.

24. C. Gilligan, *In a Different Voice* (Cambridge, Mass.: Harvard University Press, 1982), 166.

25. Gilligan, *In a Different Voice*, 62.

26. Gilligan, *In a Different Voice*, 100.

27. C. Gilligan, Moral Orientation and Moral Development, in *Women and Moral Theory*, ed. E.F. Kittay and D.T. Meyers (Totowa, N.J.: Rowan & Littlefield, 1987), 24.

28. M. Buber, *I and Thou*. New York: Scribner, 1970..

29. A. Onery, Moral Development: A Different Evaluation of Dominant Models, *Advances in Nursing Science* 6, no. 1 (1983):1–17.

30. R. Yarling and B. McElmurry, The Moral Foundations of Nursing, *Advances in Nursing Science* 8, no. 2 (1986): 63–73.

31. Bartholome, Revolution in Understanding, 10.

32. A. S. Levine, The Influence of Social and Cultural Evolution on the Relation between Professional and Patient, in *Change: A Conference on the Future of Nursing*, NIH Publication No. 81–2312 (Washington, D.C.: National Institutes of Health, 1981), 13–18.

9

Engaging the Patient: The Meaning of Illness

LISTENING TO THE STORY

Nurses are socialized by shift report and educational training to tell patient stories. Chief complaint, day and time of admission, defining physical characteristics, previous history, precipitating events, treatment plan, response to treatment, medications, and more are all part of the narrative we pass on.

All of us have our own story, a narrative that we record in our inner voice that connects events in our lives in ways that give our lives some coherence and meaning. This story is known only to us and those who are close to us. Only in times of crisis or triumph does anyone care to ask us to tell our story. When we do tell it, it comes loaded with cues and nuances that reflect the way we perceive ourselves in the world. The language we use—the "self-talk"—has meanings that have power over us but may have little impact on the casual listener.

Case managers need to be tuned in to listen and help interpret the meaning of patient stories if they are to assist the patient and other providers to discover a treatment plan that fits with the patient's spoken and unspoken needs and desires and truest sense of self. Only such a plan can motivate the patient to follow the prescribed treatment and cope with the difficult days and the pain. The care plan must be congruent with the meaning of that patient's own life.

INTERVIEWING THE PATIENT

The initial patient interview establishes the relationship between the case manager and the patient and family. It is also the beginning of an unwritten contract. The case manager identifies him- or herself, discusses his or her purpose of involvement, clarifies his or her own expectations and those of the patient, and sets a tone for the interview. The forms collecting routine information give the case manager a chance to observe the patient's response to the situation.

Most patients have a set story they give to health providers about what happened to them and how they got to the point where they are on the day of the interview. This story recounts the patient's lived experience of his or her illness. It is rich with clues to the patient's ability to cope with his or her life and illness. It contains information on his or her thoughts, cultural background, hopes for the future, self-concept, and coping style. The case manager needs the training and empathy to listen for this information because it will be important in constructing the treatment plan that has the best chance of working.

In his book *The Illness Narratives: Suffering, Healing and the Human Condition*, psychiatrist Arthur Kleinman decried the prominence of the voice of medicine over the voice of the patient's experience (life world):

> The voice of medicine drowns out the voice of the life world, often in ways that seem disrespectful, even intolerant, of the patient's perspective. . . . When the empowerment of patients and their families becomes an objective of care, the empathic auditing of their stories of the illness must be one of the clinician's chief therapeutic tasks.[1]

Kleinman was, of course, suggesting that physicians get involved in the listening process, something that many physicians have shown themselves unwilling or unable to do. Doctors are well known for interrupting patients during interviews and disregarding information that the patient feels is important. By disregarding the subjective experience of the patient, doctors have all but abandoned the role of moral agent as they treat the patient. This is particularly the case with chronically ill patients. The relational dynamic that results further alienates the patient from those in the health care system, causing increased anxiety, depression, loss of confidence, and noncompliant behavior.

Kleinman suggested that the clinician elicit a brief life history from the patient and family to sketch major events and changes in attitude, personality, major life goals, and relevant earlier experiences in coping with illness and other serious conditions. The clinician should then ask the patient to state what he or she thinks is causing the problem, when the symptoms occur and abate, and how the patient and family feel about risk, vulnerability, compliance, and satisfaction with the care received. These discussions are just the beginning. Since the patient and family narratives may be confused and confusing because of the emotional turmoil that accompanies illness, the clinician needs to check with the patient by sharing his or her understanding of the explanatory model of the patient and how it coheres with the practitioner's model. This effort is the start of a negotiated treatment plan.

The philosopher S. K. Toombs similarly stressed the need to bring together the often widely differing perspectives of patients and practitioners through mutual exploration. Toombs asserted that it is essential for doctors to consider the patient's unique range of perception, interests, knowledge, and experience that makes up his or her life story. The social meanings of the illness event that are influenced by cultural and ethnic backgrounds need full expression as the patient attempts to convey the experience of illness and the effect it has on his or her life.[2]

NEUROLINGUISTIC PROGRAMMING

The narrative that the patient shares about his or her illness is first articulated in his or her inner voice, or self-talk. Self-talk is made up of neurological events that have sensory connections. We commonly call them thoughts. Thoughts can be evoked by our conscious intention to elicit them, or, more frequently, they can be brought to consciousness by sensory input connected to past experiences. These thoughts then are "anchored" to a conditioned stimulus that evokes the same response each time we are exposed to the stimulus. Because of the anchor, a stimulus or set of stimuli will cause us to respond automatically in a certain way. This is how advertisers sell us things we do not really need.

Our specific pattern of thoughts, anchors, and reinforced stimuli gives rise to beliefs, or neurologically coded patterns of thoughts that contain specific sensory experiences of some real or imagined event. The case manager needs to discover clues to what behavioral sequences occur with each individual patient and make use of this information to connect with the patient so as to reinterpret events or bypass conscious resistance on the part of the individual.

Neurolinguistic programming was developed by Bandler and Grinder in the 1970s to describe certain linguistic patterns and neurological correlates that reveal internal thought processes.[3] According to this theory people tend to have a primary sensory modality: visual, auditory, or kinesthetic (i.e., feelings; can relate to sense of bodily position, presence, or movement resulting from the stimulation of sensorium within the body). This modality helps a person access (take in) and process (make sense of) information. People communicate using "predicates" or verbs that reflect their primary sensory modality. These can be picked out as the patient tells his or her story or recognized by other clues, such as the patient's occupation. People also reveal their primary modality through characteristic bodily signs, such as certain patterns of eye movement or speech (see Exhibit 9–1).

Not all people's sensory preferences are obvious. We all use some of the styles some of the time, and styles differ given differing circumstances. Most people can operate or freely communicate using a mix of modalities but tend to revert to their prominent mode when under stress. Preference of mode is thought to be a combination of inherited characteristics and developmental experiences.[4]

The case manager needs to speak with predicates that are congruent with the patient's individual style. The case manager can log the predicates that a person uses and then begin to use those same kinds of sensory descriptions and physical behaviors in order to build rapport with the patient. Patients will feel that they are being understood if they are matched and mirrored in this way, and may appear or act frustrated when

---

Exhibit 9–1 Sensory Modalities and Their Associated Predicates and Behaviors

	Visual	Auditory	Kinesthetic
Predicates	See, observe, look, perceive	Hear, tell, listen, sounds like	Feel, arouse, sore spot, gut feeling
Eye access	Eyes to heaven or straight ahead	Side-to-side motion when listening, look to nondominant hand	Look to dominant hand
Breathing	Shallow thoracic	Even, prolonged expiration	Deep abdominal breathing
Speech	Quick bursts of words, high nasal voice or strained tone	Clear, midrange tone, well-enunciated words	Slow, low volume or deep tone, long pauses

they are not. Additional body stances and gestures that may be culturally specific will enhance the communication between interviewer and patient.

Neurolinguistic programming has been used by psychotherapists to build rapport with patients and enhance communication between families and couples. The process of matching communication styles, or bridging the communications gap, enables therapists to anchor new responses to old events in a way that allows the events to be reinterpreted by patients.[5]

REVIEW OF ILLNESS MEANINGS

After establishing rapport with a patient, the case manager needs to discover the meaning of the illness in the patient's own story. The direct question is: How does this affect your life? Often the patient will voice feelings of frustration in the question "Why me?" The answer may be whatever the patient comes to believe is the answer. That is, there may be no inherent meaning in the illness event, only the meaning that we place there. On the face of it, most illness meanings have to do with loss. Exhibit 9–2 is a list of culturally embedded illness meanings.

According to Arthur Kleinman, there are four levels of illness meaning (see Exhibit 9–3).[6] The first level is *symptom symbols*. Kleinman stated that much meaning is stamped into body processes and that many cultural idioms reflect our tendency to symbolize emotional events and reactions in bodily terms. Physical and emotional processes are so intertwined that the person who describes daily hassles as a "pain in the neck" may well begin to experience neck pain physically. Eastern societies tend to express this interconnection by describing the body as a microcosm of symbolic reso-

---

Exhibit 9–2 Meanings and Responses to Illness Events

- *Loss*—of body image, confidence, self-concept, functional abilities, control, freedom to act, certainty, familiar world, quality of life
- *Deserved loss (punishment)*—for past behavior, real or imagined; may be embedded in religious or cultural guilt
- *Weakness*—character flaw, or overt loss of strength in face of illness
- *Enemy to be resisted*—one must fight disease process or fight those involved in treatment or care
- *Challenge to overcome the threat of loss*—motivation to recover or be healed
- *Strategy to defeat loss*—a game in which disease is cured by the performance of certain acts or strategies
- *Relief (welcomed loss)*—illness brings person to life's end, is seen as a reason to give up struggling

Exhibit 9-3 Kleinman's Four Levels of Illness Meaning

Level of Meaning	How Meanings Are Expressed
1. Symptom symbols	Body disorders suggest meanings based on cultural idiom. Body may express emotional distress via malfunctioning processes.
2. Cultural marking of disorders	The culture charges certain disorders—e.g., mental illness, leprosy, cancer, ulcers—with larger psychological or moral meanings.
3. Patient/family explanatory models	Loss and other meanings are woven into a personal mythological life narrative that reaffirms core cultural values and reintegrates the patient into society. Truths of fact are not important.
4. Clinical models	Clinical practitioners impose their own pathology-focused interpretations on the patient. The patient tends to act out stereotypes as cued by clinicians.

nance in a larger microcosm. If the body is ill, it is in disharmony. The healer's task is to bring harmony.

The second level of meaning is the *cultural marking of disorders*. Certain illnesses, such as AIDS and cancer, are charged with cultural beliefs—for example, beliefs associating the illness with flaws of character. Such beliefs leave the patient even more isolated and devoid of meaning than the illness would otherwise cause him or her to feel.

The third level of meaning is the personal and interpersonal significance that the patient and his or her family confer upon the illness experience. According to Kleinman, this level of illness meaning is clinically the most important. Patients ruminate and mull over their lives in an attempt to fit their illness into their life story and give it meaning and coherence. They look for validation of their lives and of their interpretation of the illness in order to affirm their value as human beings.

With the elderly, the stories woven become soliloquies. The recitation of the story can take on a mythical character, affirming the core cultural values of the individual and how he or she sees the self in the world. The person is thus able to reintegrate his or her social actions in a way that will enable him or her to enhance the meaning of his or her life. Those who are not able to rehearse their story to others so as to give the illness event meaning are prone to exhaustion and disillusionment. Those who continue to hope for a cure in the face of old age and chronic disease are particularly vulnerable.

The fourth level of meaning for Kleinman is clinical interpretation. The values and judgments of physicians and other health providers, and the selective listening and stereotyping in which they engage, often get in the way of helping the patient cope with chronic disease. Although the clinician may be correct about the pathology, ignoring the meaning will cause him or her to lose touch with the patient.

Toombs urged physicians to set aside their theoretical disease constructs and focus on the illness as lived by the patient—that is, to address the suffering more directly. The "healing function" is to relieve lived body disruption caused by illness. The self-perceived integrity of the patient as a person can only be restored by addressing the issue of the loss of the whole web of interrelationships of body, self, and world, especially when the illness is chronic or incurable.[7]

HEALING VERSUS CURING

If we realize that most of the situations that case managers encounter with patients have little to do with curing, we can focus our full attention on the healing aspect of case management efforts. As more people live to the stage of being frail elderly, and as there is more articulation of the value of caring over curing,[8] there is an emerging redefinition of healing in Western consciousness. Women and nurses have a special contribution to make here, as they have accepted and practiced the skills and behaviors of caring.

Jeanne Achterberg, writing about the role of women healers, defined healing as follows:

1. Healing is a lifelong journey toward wholeness.
2. Healing is remembering what has been forgotten about connection, unity and interdependence among all living and nonliving things.
3. Healing is embracing what is most feared.
4. Healing is opening what has been closed, softening what has hardened into obstruction.
5. Healing is entering the transcendent, timeless moment when one experiences the divine.
6. Healing is creativity and passion and love.
7. Healing is seeking and expressing self in its fullness, its light and shadow, male and female.
8. Healing is learning to trust life.[9]

Achterberg proposed that the full expression of health is dependent on a web that connects individuals, to each other and to a sustaining environment. This web is similar to the interdependency that according to Gilligan (Chapter 8) motivates people to behave ethically. The forms of connection are invisible and nonmaterial: they include conscious and unconscious thought, motivation, love, and will.

Achterberg saw illness and healing as existing on a number of different levels—physical, psychological, interpersonal, global, and transpersonal/ spiritual (see Figure 9–1). Although the levels are all connected, illness manifesting at a certain level demands attention and treatment specifically directed toward that level. All levels are of equal importance:

> The lessons, message and meaning of disease may relate to under-standings and accepting genetic structures inherited from one's parents, to lifestyle issues, or to more esoteric concerns. All are equally valid, equally sacred, and deserve equal recognition in a balanced approach to health.[10]

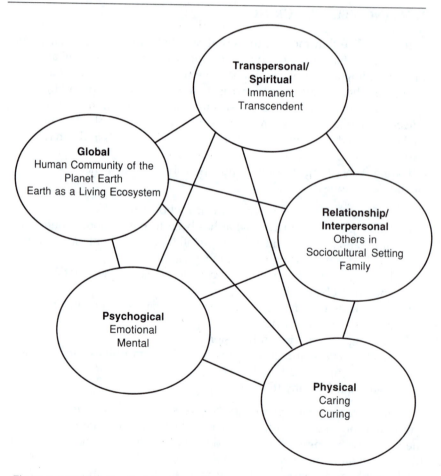

Figure 9–1 The Healing System. *Source*: From *Woman as Healer* by J. Achterberg, © 1990. Reprinted by arrangement with Shambhala Publications, Inc., 300 Massachusetts Avenue, Boston, MA 02115.

USING THE PATIENT'S EXPLANATORY MODEL TO CONSTRUCT A TREATMENT PLAN

This book assumes that the patients in contact with case managers have unique or difficult problems, which is why they were referred to case management. In many of these instances, the physician providers have already given up on the patient or have been otherwise unable to keep the plan of care focused and progressive. Therefore, the case manager is acting in a role usually thought to be reserved for physicians. Nurses often have a great deal of practice with this role because so many doctors have largely abrogated it.

After the case manager elicits the patient's story and explanatory model and gives feedback concerning how the patient's model and the case manager's model fit, the task remains for the plan of care to be negotiated between the patient and the medical providers, with the case manager as arbiter. (When we say *arbiter* here, we mean that the case manager is not the judge, but a person who knows the system, who is expected to navigate the patient through the illness event and to ensure that the process is fair.) One useful technique for this negotiation is the "SPIN" method (Story-Problem-Implication-Need; see Figure 9–2). This method was developed by consultants for large sales organizations that market goods and services requiring complex decision making and investments of time and large

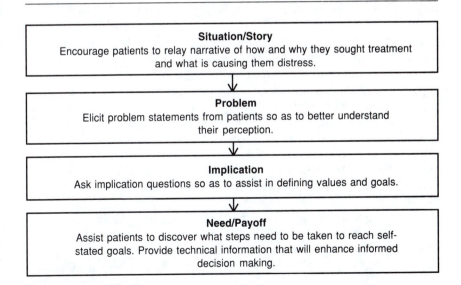

Situation/Story
Encourage patients to relay narrative of how and why they sought treatment and what is causing them distress.

↓

Problem
Elicit problem statements from patients so as to better understand their perception.

↓

Implication
Ask implication questions so as to assist in defining values and goals.

↓

Need/Payoff
Assist patients to discover what steps need to be taken to reach self-stated goals. Provide technical information that will enhance informed decision making.

Figure 9–2 The SPIN Method. *Source:* Adapted from *SPIN Selling* by N. Rackham, p. 92, with permission of Huwaite, Inc., © 1988.

amounts of money.[11] The central premise is that the marketing representative builds a relationship that leads to a sale by focusing on how the customer articulates his or her problems, exploring the implications of those problems, and through this process discovering what the customer needs.

We have already completed the first step of the SPIN method and set the stage for negotiating the treatment plan by asking the patient and family to tell the *story* of their situation in a way that reveals as complete a picture as possible concerning all the aspects of the illness. We are thus on the right track in respect to QI theory, which mandates that we regard user-defined utilities as the measure of the efficacy of our outcomes. True patient-defined (and to a lesser extent, family-defined) outcomes often have little to do with medical or even disease states. They have to do with functional, role, and life mission issues. If these issues can be resolved, healing can take place. This perspective recognizes the wholeness of the experience of being alive as a human being, not simply the dimension of health or illness.

In the second step, we ask for *problem* statements, or the patient's and family's articulation of the problems that the disease presents. This discussion leads to the third step, considering the *implications* of those problems: How in fact, does the disease affect the functioning of the patient's daily life, his or her role in the family, and his or her goals? The implication statements are the key to case management. If there is no cure for the disease and no hope to regain full functioning, then what areas of the patient's life are most affected, and in what other ways can his or her goals be met?

Implication statements concerning the degree to which sickness changes the patient's and the family's life articulate perspectives that change over time as the patient/family attempts to think through and deal with what is happening. The four stages of the dying process (disbelief, anger, bargaining, acceptance) also apply to the way most people cope with functional losses. The patient and family need to be apprised of realistic outcomes for various interventions, and they need assistance in sorting out which course to take with respect to their own values. Once the issue of values arises, patients may need time to think about how they feel or what they value. The case manager may need to come back another time to continue the discussion.

The last step is discussion of *need-payoff* questions. These questions concern what steps need to be taken to reach the patient's self-stated goals and the value of the proposed solutions in terms of how the patient and family perceive and value life and quality of life, how much they trust technological interventions, and how they evaluate risk and longevity. The endpoint is that the patient proposes the treatment plan/solution on the basis of his or her perception of the problems, the implications of those problems, and his or her values. At the point that the patient can articulate the benefits of the proposed care plan, the case manager is aware of the level of commitment and motivation to follow the agreed-upon course of action.

The case manager then writes up the plan while checking with the patient as to whether all of his or her concerns have been covered. The benefits of the care plan are reviewed and summarized. The patient and family are asked to make an appropriate level of commitment. For very difficult patients, this may involve a patient contract (see Chapter 10).

DECISION STYLES

Decision-making styles of patients and their families are an important consideration in the negotiation of the treatment plan. Generally speaking, the older the patient, the more likely it is that the patient will give his or her decision making over to the physician.[12] A study by Pierce that used a survey method to classify decision-making styles of women deciding on breast cancer treatment found that younger patients seemed willing to take more risks and more personal responsibility for their decisions than older patients (see Table 9–1).[13] Pierce described them as "deliberators": they tended to consider various risks explicitly, use a mental strategy that identified attributes of each alternative, and gather specific information about each treatment option. Although the deliberators expressed less confidence than the more passive decision makers, they also gave more consideration to each treatment option. Pierce called their decision rule the "last-difference rule"—a decision was made only after information on all alternatives was reviewed.

In reference to the case manager's involvement in patient decision making, Cody argued that the term *manager* is not congruent with the principle of autonomy afforded adults in health decision making. The patient should be the case manager, he stated.[14] No good case manager would argue with this view. Case managers who wish to have the best patient-defined outcome will assist patients with the information-gathering and decision-making process so that patients can arrive at the best outcome for them.

LIFE EXTENSION ISSUES

The issue of life extension seems to be injecting itself more regularly into public discussion. Whether we feel that Dr. Kevorkian is a criminal or a merciful hero in the 20-plus suicides he has assisted, there is no doubt that

Table 9–1 Decision-Making Styles of Women Deciding on Breast Cancer Treatment

Decision Style	Salience of Alternatives	Conflict	Information Seeking	Risk Awareness	Deliberation	Decision Rule
Deferrer N = 20 (41%) M age = 56 years	Immediate attraction to one option	None	None	Risk-averse	None	Simple preference
Delayer N = 21 (44%) M age = 45 years	Considers at least two options	Yes minimal	Minimal (prefers non-technical sources)	Risk-averse	Vacillation	"First difference"
Deliberator N = 7 (15%) M age = 40 years	Considers and decomposes at least two options	Yes moderate	Extensive (prefers technical sources)	Risk-seeking	Strategy	"Last difference"

Source: Reprinted from Pierce, P.F., Deciding on Breast Cancer Treatment: A Description of Decision Behavior, *Nursing Research*, Vol. 42, No. 1, p. 24, with permission of the American Journal of Nursing Co., © 1993.

people are questioning the never-say-die medical model.[15] Decisions by teenagers to forgo chemotherapy treatment and immunosuppressive medication are also breaking up the usual ways of thinking about longevity versus quality of life.[16]

As many people are living longer, it appears that the money to care for them under the present system will become increasingly limited. According to Daniel Callahan, "Contemporary moral philosophy shows considerable nervousness about extending the scope of moral obligation much beyond explicitly understood and accepted contractual agreements."[17] Perhaps this is because the justice perspective on ethics cannot speak adequately to this issue. For Callahan, there is something incongruous about the medical system's push to extend treatment without limits for human beings whose nature it is to age and die.[18] In his view, medical goals for life extension should not be pursued, since the costs are high and the benefit to society as a whole is slight. Elder advocates should work toward the development of an integrated perspective of a natural life span. Further, our society should alter its perception of death as an enemy to be held off at all costs and consider it instead as a condition of life to be accepted, "if not for its own sake, then for the sake of others."[19] In response to the problem of an increasingly expensive Medicare entitlement program, Callahan proposed a Medicare "Part C," in which the elderly could choose a restriction on hospital benefits and receive enhanced quality-of-life benefits in return.[20]

Case managers are faced with difficult issues, and end-of-life decisions are among the most perplexing. Medically marginal, unlikely, or futile treatments (with over 20%, 7 to 20%, or under 7% of patients responding to treatment, respectively) do nothing but drive up the cost of care and decrease the patient's quality of life. Moreover, they divert the patient and family from dealing with personal issues that are laden with meaning. Death is indeed tragic if we are not afforded the opportunity to cope with these issues before death takes place.

NOTES

1. A. Kleinman, *The Illness Narratives: Suffering, Healing and the Human Condition* (New York: Basic Books, 1988), 230.

2. S.K. Toombs, *The Meaning of Illness: A Phenomenological Account of the Different Perspectives of the Patient and Physician* (Boston: Klewer Academic Press, 1993), 26–27.

3. R. Bandler and J. Grinder, *The Structure of Magic*, vol. 1 (Palo Alto, Calif.: Science and Behavior Books, 1975).

4. D. Brockopp, What Is NLP? *American Journal of Nursing* (1983):1012–1014.

5. S. Davis and D. Davis, *Neurolinguistic Programming and Family Therapy*, 9 (1983):283–291.

6. Kleinman, *Illness Narratives*, 233.

7. Toombs, *Meaning of Illness*, 115–117.

8. S. Nuland, *How We Die* (1994). New York: Knopf.

9. J. Achterberg, *Woman as Healer* (Boston: Shambhala Press, 1990), 194.

10. Achterberg, *Woman as Healer*, 195–196.

11. N. Rackham, *SPIN Selling* (New York: McGraw-Hill, 1988).

12. A. Beisecker, Aging and the Desire for Information and Input in Medical Decisions, *The Gerontologist* 28 (1988):330–335.

13. P.F. Pierce, Deciding on Breast Cancer Treatment: A Description of Decision Behavior, *Nursing Research* 42, no. 1 (1993):22–27.

14. W.K. Cody, Radical Health-Care Reform: The Person as Case Manager, *Nursing Science Quarterly* 7, no. 4 (1994):180–182.

15. C. Mayer, At Trial, a Chorus of Women Is Voicing Support for Dr. Kevorkian, *Philadelphia Inquirer*, 29 April 1994, A-21.

16. "Behind a Boy's Decision to Forgo Treatment," *New York Times*, 13 June 1994, A-8.

17. D. Callahan, *Setting Limits: Medical Goals in an Aging Society* (New York: Simon & Shuster, Inc., 1987), 102.

18. Callahan, *Setting Limits*, 203.

19. Callahan, *Setting Limits*, 223.

20. D. Callahan, High Tech or Long Term Care? Let the Elderly Decide, *New York Times*, 12 June 1994, H-12.

10

Patient-Centered
Goal Setting

༄༅

Once the case manager has established a level of communication with
the patient and family that enables him or her to know the implications of
the illness and patient- and family-defined needs and wants, an appropriate care plan can be constructed. This chapter concerns step-by-step
techniques in goal setting and strategies for actually reaching goals.

PERSONALIZING GOALS

When we know how an illness affects a person's daily routine and
quality of life, we have gained some insight into what he or she values. If
the patient and family have some difficulty articulating the illness's effects, we may want to spend some time having them articulate their values.
The following steps are recommended.

First, the patient and family members each make a list of their personal
values. The list should be broken down into dimensions of everyday life:
physical functioning and health, mental and emotional well-being, family
and home environment, spiritual and ethical life, financial condition, and
social and cultural environment. Each of these dimensions is affected
when a person or a family member is ill. Then each person prioritizes
values by importance and describes his or her individual goals in reference
to the values listed.

The information that emerges from this exercise can have a major impact on how patient and family members perceive the illness event and what their individual roles are during the evolving crisis. For example, many gravely ill people tend to ruminate and get depressed over financial issues, or who is going to take care of the dog when they are gone. These issues may not be seen as real at all to other members of the family, even the spouse. When they get put on the table, such fears tend not to be as troubling as they were when no one would acknowledge their existence. Much of the patient's anxiety seems to melt away.

The next step is to look at how the goals in each real-life domain are connected to the patient-articulated meaning of illness. Here again, the results can be quite unexpected. The sharing that goes on between family members and the case manager sets the tone for honest communication concerning needs and obligations and defines the level of commitment among members of the family, thus encouraging a sense of self-responsibility (see Case Example).

Case Example

George was a 49-year-old white male who was admitted to the hospital for diagnostic studies. He complained of diffuse abdominal pain that was similar to pain he had experienced for many years, but was now worse. He was subsequently diagnosed with stomach cancer which had also metastasized to the liver. George took this as a death sentence and was depressed. The depressive symptoms seemed to exacerbate his pain. The family doctor asked a nurse case manager to see George.

George was the chief of maintenance of the hospital where the case manager was employed. Since it was a community hospital many employees had learned of George's condition. George grew up and learned his trade under the tutelage of an overbearing father who forced him to work in a variety of building trades from a very young age. George resented his lost childhood, the long hours which he subsequently worked, and the lack of family life that ensued as he rose, without a high school education, from an entry level position in the hospital maintenance department to the head of the department.

George believed that he was able to rise to that position because he knew so much about every aspect of building construction and maintenance from his experience with his father. However, he still resented the hardship he perceived that his father had forced him to bear.

The case manager did an extensive interview with the patient, and found that George had been having abdominal pain for many years, but chose to ignore it. "My anger with my father was eating me up, but I had to work harder than anyone else if I was going to survive and feed my family." George actually had very few signs of illness other than the pain. He had not lost his appetite or any weight. He was unable to function at his job because of the emotional distress. He felt unable to discuss his situation with his wife. He avoided discussing his illness with his children. The case manager drew up a list of categories and worked with George to identify those that were most distressing, as seen in Exhibit 10–1.

The case manager worked with George to identify problems in each area of his life and prioritize the severity of the perceived problems. Then she went to his home and sat with his wife and children (ages 11, 14, and 15) to facilitate their understanding of the issues George was facing and to assist them in articulating the important family issues. The case manager's efforts resulted in a change in George's behavior in the following ways:

1. George was able to go back to work and assume the duties of his position. He began to train the assistant department head to assume more responsibility so that he could take over the department in the future.
2. George began to go home at 5 p.m. for the first time in his life.
3. Because he was home for dinner, George was introduced to his children in a way he had never before experienced.
4. He realized that he had been acting out a life similar to his father's, even while he resented his father's life patterns.
5. He took time to seek pastoral counseling at his church, and received additional counseling from a psychologist to sort out his feelings and anger toward his father.
6. George discovered that he also held much anger which was directed at himself, as he felt helpless to have a more normal family life in the past.

In the hospital, everyone waits for the captain of the ship (the attending physician) to discuss the patient's condition with the patient and family so that treatment decisions can be made. When the doctor does not face the issue and procrastinates, it sets up frustration between the patient/family and the hospital staff, particularly the nurses, who are left to hear the complaints. The issue of self-responsibility is not dealt with because the

Exhibit 10–1 Goal-Setting for George

Problem Area	Long-Term Goals	Short-Term Goals	Action Steps
Terminal diagnosis of cancer	Live as long as it takes to achieve goals	1. Full review of treatment options 2. Treatment course which will allow George to remain active and working	1. Referral to oncologist who is willing to work with George's wish to remain working during treatment 2. Schedule sick/vacation time to accommodate treatment regimen
Depression	To be free of symptoms which prevent George from working and coping with treatment regimen	1. To discover things to feel good about in daily life 2. To learn to induce positive feeling or at least a relaxed state for ten minutes three times per day	1. Seek counseling assistance to do life inventory with a focus on positive accomplishments George has made in his life, and to identify new goals 2. To learn relaxation exercises that George feels comfortable doing 3. To plan the best place and time for George to take time for himself each day to perform his exercises
Problems with job	To be able to function effectively at work for as long as possible	1. To cope with demands of job on a daily basis 2. To delegate responsibilities and train subordinates to take over various responsibilities	1. Speak with VP of operations to inform him of circumstance and plans to train subordinates and gradually relinquish control 2. Ask VP for assistance in planning and carrying out plans 3. Identify sources of assistance and ask for help as needed

Family	To minimize distress to wife and children	1. Approach each day with a clear plan and the attitude to achieve long term goal	1. Make time for family as a whole and wife and each child individually 2. Enter family counseling so that feelings can be discussed by entire family
Financial problems	Family will be without financial difficulties	1. Identify short-term and long-term needs of family	1. Engage financial counselor to review insurance and current financial state 2. Carry out recommendations as suggested
Spiritual distress	To reach a mental and emotional state where the prospect of death is not anxiety provoking	1. Goals same as with depression 2. Renew church-going habits to induce a "state of grace"	1. Find a priest that George feels comfortable with discussing his problems 2. Make time for spiritual exercises/prayers each day

doctor has set the moral tone by his own lack of responsibility. Conversely, practitioners who address issues head on are helping patients and families to direct their own attention and energy to the real issues and are providing an opportunity for healing to take place.

MAKING THE GOALS REAL

Now that the patient and family have prioritized their goals in terms of their values, they can take steps to make the goals real. These goals need to seem attainable, and the only way to make them attainable is to make them seem progressively more real as they are developed and as steps are taken to attain them.

As the patient and family focus on solutions, the magnitude of the problems tends to diminish. Solution-focused thinking and acting give the patient and family a sense of control over the situation. Patients can more easily separate themselves from the situation, holding onto positive attitudes that will enhance the possibility of success. Focusing on goals helps keep things in perspective, enabling patients to keep up with their therapeutic regime and enabling more positive and timely decision making.

Goal statements are constructed by addressing questions in the following sequence:

1. Where do we stand now?
2. What are our priorities?
3. What does the solution look like? The solution is built into a picture that is explored during daily visualization exercises.
4. What does the solution feel like? What sensations do I have as the goal is achieved?
5. What sounds do I hear when the goal is achieved? What are the ambient sounds present once I have achieved the goals? (Are there birds singing in the background as I relax in my favorite chair and see the sunset?) What do other people say to me as I am achieving my goals?

Goal statements cannot be constructed overnight. It takes practice, assistance, and perseverance to set goals, anchor them to one's sensory life, and construct the details of the desired endpoint. As the goals are being constructed in the patient's mind, a plan of action becomes evident. The details of the goals suggest what steps need to be taken and the time frames for taking them. The steps themselves are broken down into manageable tasks that can be practiced until small successes are achieved. Measures of meeting the goals, determined by the patient in advance, will provide confirmation that a goal is achieved (see Exhibit 10–2).

Obstacles are considered separately. The focus must be on the positive, and some obstacles that are initially present may subside as the goal statements become more clear. Obstacles are issues that others besides the patient can often attend to. There is no point in letting the patient become involved in obsessing over obstacles.

Affirmations are positive statements that are repeated a number of times a day so that goal statements can become more real. They are formulated in the following way:

1. Identify goals/areas of functional or well-being improvement.
2. Identify benefits to be gained once a goal is achieved.
3. Write a trial affirmation. Affirmations are written in the first person ("I"), use the present tense, are always stated positively (i.e., the word *no* or *not* is never used), and should be fun or enjoyable.
4. The affirmation is tested and refined as to how well it follows the above rules.[1]
5. The affirmation is repeated at regular intervals during periods of "readiness."[2]

Affirmations that will assist the patient to visualize and maintain motivation to achieve the goals need to be internalized and become part of the person's self-talk. Therefore, the patient must be ready to accept the goals/affirmations. Readiness is a function of willingness and ability. If the patient is willing to change, his or her ability to change is contingent on the ability to accept new information and messages that will challenge his or her previous ideas and self-talk.

Readiness is enhanced when affirmations are repeated to a consciousness that is not troubled. The patient must be in a relaxed, pain-free frame of mind, with no distractions that will disable the messages. The affirmations will then be able to replace the old messages, fears, and anxieties with messages that become more real with each repetition. Thus, the self-talk of the patient is moving toward an outcome that the patient has defined and continues to define as he or she constructs the anchors (pictures, feelings, and sounds) that make the goals more real to him or her.

MAKING THE GOALS POSITIVE

The goal statements should be reviewed against the criteria used to set them up: How are they congruent with the patient's goals concerning

Exhibit 10–2 Goal-setting Worksheet for Chronically Ill People

Domain/Problem	Short-Term Goal	Action Steps	Measure of Meeting Goal (circle on 5-point scale 1 = Best 5 = Worst)	Long-Term Goal
Loss of function	Reduce, eliminate, or adapt to disabling effects of disorder	1. 2. 3.	1 2 3 4 5	Optimal ADLs
Loss of body image	Decrease emotional distress	1. 2.	1 2 3 4 5	Acceptance/change in attitudes/beliefs
Psychic/spiritual distress	Feel good at least 10 minutes 3 times per day	1. 2. 3.	1 2 3 4 5	Positive feeling state
Problems with family	Improve communication	1. 2.	1 2 3 4 5	Coping/closure
Problems with job		1. 2.	1 2 3 4 5	Adaptation
Side effects of therapy	Identify cause Provide relief	1. 2. 1. 2.	1 2 3 4 5	Complete therapy, minimize side effects
Other		1.	1 2 3 4 5	

Note: This worksheet can be used by patients, family members, case managers, and other providers as appropriate. Compare scores and revise periodically as needed.

functional health, quality of life, spiritual life, family life, financial condition, and social life? Goals that are unrealistic and not life affirming will not develop in the patient's consciousness to become real. What is important to that patient, whether acknowledged to self and others or not, will make itself known to the patient's consciousness if the above technique is consistently followed. Thus, as the plan of care evolves, the goals of the patient, the goals of the family, and the natural course of healing converge. By affirming his or her life goals through statements and short- and longer term objectives, the patient is *healing him- or herself*. The patient gets a glimpse of how to connect with what and who is really important in his or her life and what things he or she must do to achieve the experience of wholeness.

CHANGING BEHAVIORS

By changing the habits of thought and directing the attention of patients and families to make goals real through visualization and affirmation, the case manager has already begun to change behaviors. This process continues as patient and family take the steps articulated in the goals to the actual goal attainment. Continuing reinforcement of motivation can be supplied by continuing use of visualization and affirmation, social support, and the steady achievement of small successes.

Exhibit 10–3 summarizes the steps of setting and achieving goals.

Exhibit 10–3 Steps in Setting and Achieving Goals

1. Do self-evaluation and set priorities based on own values.
2. Use "I want/I wish" statements to practice building goals.
3. Fill in details of plan and set deadlines.
4. List things most easily achieved first.
5. Prejudge worthiness of a goal and ability to meet it.
6. Enhance desire by visualization and affirmations. Repeat visualization/affirmation exercise at spaced intervals throughout the day after inducing readiness through relaxation techniques.
7. Build confidence by achieving small goals and by learning new ways to achieve goals.
8. Enhance determination by repeating goals and reality checking with others. Elicit social support as needed.

STRESS INOCULATION TECHNIQUES

Stress inoculation techniques (SIT) are cognitive–behavioral techniques that use counseling, coaching, and a repertoire of interventions to enable patients/clients to cope successfully with stress.[3] SIT theory assumes that stress is a result of a transaction between person and environment, influenced by both the environmental stimuli and the appraisal of events by the person. Stress is a cognitively mediated relational concept that exists in tension between possible positive or negative anticipated outcomes. Events that are perceived as stressful will in fact be stressful. Those that can be perceived in less threatening ways can more easily be coped with. Thus, SIT "inoculates" a person against the debilitating effects of possible stressful events.

According to SIT theory, stressed individuals inadvertently create and engender reactions in others that maintain maladaptive stress responses. Stress inoculation techniques enlist patients and clients as collaborators in collecting data that lead to their recognizing low-intensity cues and learning to interrupt and change them. (See Figure 10–1).

The following are strategies used in SIT:

1. *Discussion of problem*: Patient defines the scope of the problem. Case manager establishes rapport and meaning of illness, and looks for phrases or attitudes that demonstrate that automatic thinking (negative self-talk) is taking place.
2. *Didactic teaching/Socratic questioning* to reduce negative appraisals.
3. *Cognitive restructuring*: reconceptualizing the event so as not to appear so threatening. For example, the case manager might ask, "On a scale of 1 to 100, how threatening can the worst case scenario be?" (This kind of question, when asked of patients, is the basis for the Sickness Impact Profile and other well-validated health status questionnaires.)
4. *Problem solving*: elicit suggestions from the patient. Discuss relative merits of action plan with patient and family. Use drawings and grids to write out pros and cons of treatment options.
5. *Relaxation training* to give respite from threatening appraisal and to prepare the patient to accept positive affirmations and behavioral rehearsal. Treatment should start immediately. Different people respond to different styles or techniques to induce a relaxation state.
6. *Behavioral and image rehearsal*: Patient practices coping with threatening images, assisted by someone who coaches him or her through the process.
7. *Self-monitoring*: Patient is trained at "thought catching," or recognizing the rapid thoughts, images, and feelings that occur under stress. These "automatic thoughts" can be unprompted by events and usually have specific content, such as interpretation of or predictions about situations and events. The patient can be consciously unaware

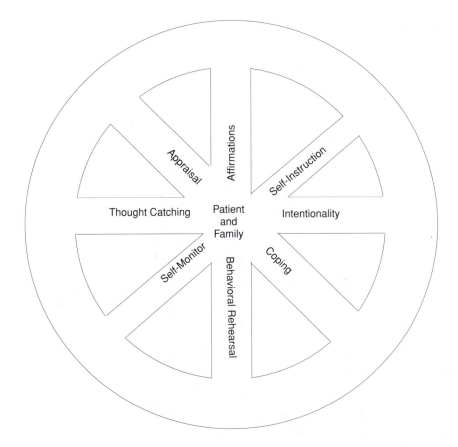

Figure 10–1 Stress Innoculation Approach To Restructuring Behavior. Things that can be done to assist patients and families to be their own case managers.

of them but respond to the content and affect they introduce (see examples in Exhibit 10–4).

8. *Self-instruction:* The patient has goals and action steps that have been formulated as part of the care plan. These include statements concerning how to focus his or her attention if his or her ability to handle stress is an identified problem.

9. *Self-reinforcement:* This includes affirmations and other techniques to change appraisal of the possible stressful events.

10. *Environmental change:* Some stressors can only be coped with by actually changing the outside source of the events (e.g., dispensing analgesics for pain, or moving to a warmer climate for patients with cardiac disease).

Exhibit 10–4 Examples of Stress-Engendering Automatic Thoughts

---
- What's the use—the therapy isn't going to work anyway.
- It's such an effort to do anything.
- Life has no meaning.
- These thoughts (or feelings) just overwhelm me.
- Life's a bitch and then you die.
- I'll probably die at 40 just like my father did.
- No one really cares for me.
- There is nothing that I can do to control this.

Source: Compiled from *Stress Inoculation Training* by D. Meichenbaum, Pergamon Press, 1985.

COACHING

When there are missteps, breakdowns, and perseverations in the patient's behavior, the case manager's coaching skills are called on. After eliciting the patient/family's interpretation of what went wrong or what performance is unsatisfactory (in terms of taking action steps set forth in the care plan), the case manager should take the following steps:

1. Get an agreement that a problem exists and define the nature of the problem.
2. Mutually discuss alternative solutions.
3. Mutually agree on action to be taken to solve the problem.
4. Follow up to ensure that the agreed action has been taken.
5. Recognize any achievement when it occurs.[4]

Successfully changing others' behavior depends on

1. identifying the desired behavioral change and the need for it
2. face-to-face involvement with the patient/family
3. a connection between patient/family behavior and results
4. the patient/family seeing that what is happening is in their own interest
5. maximized feedback to the patient/family[5]

CONTRACTING

A contract is an agreement between two or more people. Contracting is a way to formalize understandings and action steps to promote the carrying out of an agreed-upon treatment plan. It can help all parties to clarify

Exhibit 10–5 Elements of a Patient Contract

- **Assumptions**
  1. Equal power
  2. Independence
  3. Consensual relationship
  4. Willingness to negotiate
  5. Each will gain from the encounter
  6. Evolves over time
- **Responsibilities**
  1. Patient: honesty and consideration of proposed recommendations
  2. Provider: gives due diligence to discover problem and offer alternative solutions to the patient/family. Keeps current on clinical knowledge. Takes no undue risks.

goals, roles, behaviors, meanings, and motivations. This process can keep everyone focused on activities that will lead to healing.

Exhibit 10–5 sets forth the assumptions and responsibilities of those involved in the contract.[6] Exhibit 10–6 sets forth the procedural steps leading to negotiating a contract in helper relationships. Here again we find that successful contracts have the elements of autonomous and consensual relationships built on respect.[7] The contract evolves over time and is a shared-risk arrangement. Caretaker and patient are bound to each other. Honesty and due diligence on both sides are assumed.

Steps for Drawing up a Contract

Procedurally, we are negotiating the contract as we go through the steps to draw it up. Most of the routine information that provides the basis for the contract has already been gathered, and the relationship with the patient is well established by the time the subject of a contract comes up. If the parties know each other's needs and trust each other, contracts are fairly easy to negotiate. They are helpful for those with cognitive injuries and other memory loss, they bring positive changes in how families relate to each other, and they provide reinforcement for the whole treatment team to be compliant with the treatment plan (this is no small achievement!). The contract may not be signed by all members of the treatment team, but all need to be aware of it because their role will be better defined by it.

A contract is written in the following sequence:

1. The case manager meets with the patient/family and other involved parties. The care plan and roles in carrying it out are reviewed.

Exhibit 10–6 Contracting in Helping Relationships

- Introduction
  1. Nature of relationship
  2. Services helper provides
  3. Helper's background and experience
  4. Time frames and fees
  5. Expectations of the client
  6. Limits upon each one's expectations
- Clarify meanings/roles/goals
- Communicate/document
- Negotiate/reframe/coach

2. Goal statements are written.
3. A statement is written on actions to be taken to solve problems or reach goals.
4. A statement is written spelling out roles of participants.
5. A statement is included keeping the contract open to change.
6. Signatures and date are appended.

An Example of Contracting

Mary B., a 68-year-old nursing home resident with progressive weakness in her legs and some forgetfulness, had become progressively more incontinent over the last month. The fingerpointing between Mary and the nursing assistants had worsened, as she frequently denied that she needed to be toileted or refused to be toileted. The case manager in the LTC facility recognized the change in functional status and realized that the memory loss was real. She therefore initiated the following contract with the resident:

This is an agreement between resident Mary B. and nursing case manager Helen G. regarding Mary B.'s treatment.

1. Mary agrees that she does not like to be incontinent.
2. Mary agrees that she wants to walk more frequently so that she doesn't lose the ability to do so and wind up in a wheelchair for the rest of her life.
3. Mary doesn't want to have any urinary tract infections or sores on her bottom.
4. Therefore, Mary agrees to a schedule of being walked to the toilet every two hours, from wherever she is sitting, during the hours of 6 a.m. to 8 p.m. Mary will be placed on a bedpan at

night or will choose to walk to the bathroom. This will be referred to as the bowel and bladder program, or the B&B.

5. If Mary forgets the terms of this agreement, it will be shown to her, and there will be no hard feelings on anybody's part. Mary can refuse to be toileted at any time, but in full knowledge of the provisions of this agreement.

6. This agreement can be changed by negotiation of the parties.

Signatures: Resident, Case manager, Day shift charge nurse.

This statement was posted on the back of Mary's bedroom door, wheelchair high. It was also in the chart and listed in the care plan cardex. The nursing assistants all claimed this tactic would never work.

Mary would usually refuse to be toileted when she was in or near the bedroom door. Now, when she refused to be toileted, she was reminded of the contract and wheeled up to the door to read the statement and examine her signature. She would then consent to being walked to and from the bathroom. After a month, she rarely felt the need to examine the document and only had to be reminded of its existence. She continued to be continent and functional as long as the bowel and bladder program was followed.

When To Contract

Contracts can be used in many different settings. They may be used with complex cases when the treatment is fraught with complications. They may be used to challenge patients to take more responsibility for themselves and their well-being. They may be used to set boundaries for others in the treatment team or the family. Recalcitrant substance abuse patients may also respond to a contract. This only works when there is clear advantage to the patient to be compliant with the agreement. Thus, rigging the incentives is congruent with managed-care theory, if not with current practice.

Legal Implications of Contracting

The chief legal risks of contracting would arise only if one party were to act negligently after making the agreement. Then there would be little discussion over actual liability. The requirements to prove negligence are (1) duty of reasonable standard of care; (2) breach of duty by act or omission; (3) cause (but for the breach, the injury would not have occurred); and (4) injury (or damage) must be shown.[8] Patient contracts actually help prevent litigation charging negligence because more things are spelled out and there has been direct communication and trust building to reach the contract. Simply constructing the contract protects caregivers from the charge of negligence:

1. It shows that the most reasonable standards of care have been upheld through consensus on what the care plan specifies.
2. It demonstrates that steps and controls have been constructed to ensure that omissions or other breach of duty will be unlikely.
3. Because it specifies the treatment plan and makes it public, it constitutes a proactive step to lower the possibility that injury (unanticipated harm outside the disease course) will occur.
4. Any harm to the patient that does occur is thus unlikely to be a result of negligent behavior on the part of health care providers. Documentation will support this view.

TRANSFORMING THE PATIENT INTO A CASE MANAGER

We are now teaching patients and their families to take on the role of case manager. We are asking them to appraise their situation in a different way, decide what their values and goals are, perform the action steps, model and rehearse their behaviors, monitor maladaptive thoughts, and redirect the thoughts to a more positive focus based on their value system. We have been coaching and counseling patients and families to self-heal. These activities have been called *transformational leadership*. (See Figure 10–2).

Transformational leadership is leadership preparing the follower to take over the role and tasks of the leader. It leads to growth for the client and the leader and is characterized by mutuality and affiliation, acknowledgment of complexity and ambiguity, cooperation rather than competition, focus on process rather than task, networking rather than hierarchy, and recognition of the value of intuition.[9]

The case manager, by engaging the patient and family in a process of discovery and self-healing, has elevated the relationship to a different level. The patient is connected with others while remaining autonomous, and he or she can direct his or her focus away from negative appraisals so that healing has the opportunity to take place.

By establishing the patient as an autonomous person who is capable of choosing to act in ways that will assist him or her to cope, the case manager has set a tone for interaction. This tone should be kept throughout the relationship with the patient/family so as to enhance compliance with the treatment plan.

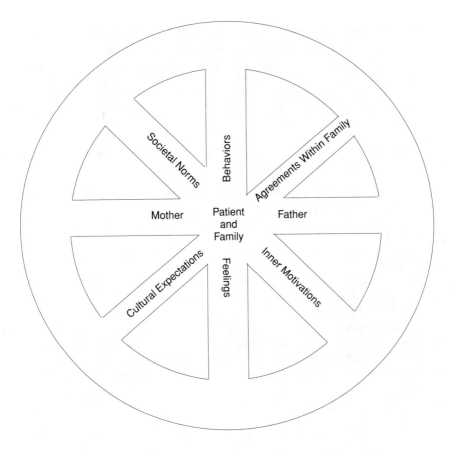

Figure 10–2 The case manager nurtures coping by modeling transactions which promote coherence and healing.

SUMMARY

We have reviewed strategies that enable us to incorporate patient-defined meanings of illness and goals into a treatment plan and to set up a framework of incentives and behaviors that will assist the patient and family to carry it out. We have done so with the full consent of the parties involved. We have taken on the challenge of changing the patient's life-long pattern of conscious and unconscious behaviors. We have set up contracts that can clarify communication, assist in problem solving, enhance good feelings, aid in goal acquisition, and provide inoculation against stress and lawsuits.

Anyone who has worked with individuals who are disabled or terminally ill and who are honestly confronting their conditions can tell stories of the courage, ingenuity, and triumph of spirit that these people manifest in their everyday lives. A patient-centered case management approach that uses processes to bring all issues to the table for discussion and problem solving is the best way to set up an opportunity for healing to take place.

NOTES

1. P.J. Meyer, *Dynamics of Personal Goal Setting* (Waco, Tex.: Success Motivation Inc., 1988).

2. E. Miller, *Immuno-Imagery* (Irvine, Calif.: Bio-Imagery, Inc., 1993).

3. The review of SIT here mostly draws on D. Meichenbaum, *Stress Inoculation Training* (New York: Pergamon Press, 1985).

4. F. Fournies, *Coaching for Improved Work Performance* (New York: Van Nostrand Reinhold, 1978).

5. Fournies, *Coaching for Improved Work Performance.*

6. T.E. Quih, Partnerships in Patient Care: A Contractual Approach. *Annals of Internal Medicine* (1983) 98:228–234.

7. S. Molde, Understanding Patients' Agendas. *Image* (1986) 4:145–147.

8. D. Slee, Negligence, in *The Law of Hospital and Health Care Administration*, 2nd. ed., ed. A. Southwick (Ann Arbor, Mich.: Hospital Administration Press, 1988), 52–100.

9. A.M. Barker, An Emerging Leadership Paradigm, *Nursing and Health Care* 12 (1991):204–207.

Part III

Engaging the Future

11

Engaging the Future: The Demedicalization of Health

Part I of this book reviewed the theories, settings, and types of nursing case management and the strategies that case managers use to manage costs and obtain resources to manage care. Part II reviewed how the case manager should engage the patient as a person who is intimately involved in his or her treatment plan; outlined techniques and tools for setting patient-defined goals incorporating the patient's meanings of illness; and set forth an ethical framework that involves the patient in the activities of caring and self-care. Part III looks at how managed care is driving technological, structural, and paradigm changes as well as the adoption of a new, broad range of humanistic clinical techniques. These changes open up new options for creative treatment plans to be discovered by the patient and the rest of the care team. Case management coordinates the process of discovery and implementation.

HOW THE HEALTH CARE DELIVERY SYSTEM IS CHANGING

Case management is changing as the health care delivery system itself is changing. Case managers demonstrate the value of their services if they understand the causes and future implications of these changes as they take place.

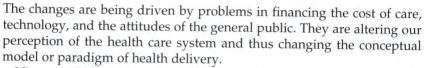

The changes are being driven by problems in financing the cost of care, technology, and the attitudes of the general public. They are altering our perception of the health care system and thus changing the conceptual model or paradigm of health delivery.

Nine paradigm shifts in health care are discussed below.

The Acute Care System Is Adapting to Chronic Care Requirements

Traditionally, the majority of patients had acute needs due to disease or injury springing from a single biological cause. The patient was a generally passive recipient of a cure. However, the dominant illness (disease plus functional and quality-of-life consequences) pattern is now chronic: that is, gradually debilitating illness stemming from multiple biopsychosocial factors (e.g., age, stress, maladaptive health habits).

Since there is no cure for chronic disease, appropriate care looks to relieve suffering and to maintain optimal physical and emotional functioning. Treatment is a continuous process that should involve techniques outside traditional allopathic medicine if these may enhance quality of life or fit with the patient's perception of need based on cultural or other beliefs. Treatment can be successful only if the patient is actively participating in his or her treatment plan. The old health care system, in which the hospital is the central focus, costs too much in dollars and quality of life. Managed-care organizations (MCOs) make sense only to the extent that they can offer an organized system of comprehensive services delivered at a fixed price. MCOs can enhance their services using case management to manage the delivery of chronic care.

The Fee-for-Service (FFS) System Is Shifting to a System of Capitation Payment (or Global Budgets)

FFS plus a large number of uninsured and below-cost reimbursements (i.e., Medicare and Medicaid) have destabilized the system. The simple change in the way MCOs pay for services converts all providers from revenue producers to cost centers. This change fundamentally threatens every provider discipline except for nursing, since nurses have almost always been cost centers. Each provider is now compelled to find ways to structure efficient, high-quality care into daily practice. The understanding and diligent application of the principles of QI and health outcomes measures will guide practitioners in adapting to the new environment.

QA is Becoming QI

The focus of quality efforts is changing from identifying and punishing provider outliers to identifying teams who will rethink work processes and reinvent service delivery on the basis of the projected outcome of care (QI). QI is an incremental system of change that may be too slow and labor intensive for some health care executives, who are uncomfortable with bottom-up process changes.

Reengineering Is Being Introduced for Rapid Process Changes

The use of information systems, including high-speed scanners, voice recognition software, hand-held computers, graphic user interfaces, real-time data retrieval, and extensive clinical/decision support databases, will revolutionize the practice of medicine and health care to a point at which it will be barely recognizable to present-day practitioners. Practice patterns, resource use, and the contract management needs of providers and payers will force large investments in information systems, not to change but to replace current processes. These large-scale process changes have huge risks as well as potential benefits.

The following is a partial list of reengineering projects that will change the process of how health care is delivered and administered:

1. Telemedicine, in which rural practitioners will be able to speak and demonstrate a patient to a tertiary care specialist via video links
2. Data glove links and telemonitoring technology so that a doctor at a remote site can see and feel what the on-site practitioner is experiencing, thus coaching and diagnosing from a remote location[1]
3. Community health information networks (CHINs) that will make health-related data on patients available at the point of service[2]
4. Voice recognition technology that will transcribe dictated reports, thus eliminating many clerical positions
5. Optical scanning and retrieval technology that will scan patient records, retrieve selected information from those records, and store vast amounts of data on laser disks for quick retrieval
6. Computerized decision support that can contain patient specific clinical paths, even paths constructed to account for multiple diagnoses

The Confidentiality of Patient Information Is Being Rethought

The current state of confidentiality in the traffic of patient records bears little resemblance to the ideal. As a committee report on regional health data networks stated, patient authorizations for the release of medical information are often not voluntary because patients feel compelled to sign the authorization or forgo the benefit sought, and are not informed because they cannot know in advance what information will be in the record, who will subsequently have access to it, and how it will be used. A new way of viewing who owns the data and how to safeguard those who may be hurt from the sharing of such data has been proposed by the Institute of Medicine.[3] The Institute of Medicine looks to health database organizations (HDOs) to link data outside the care setting so that appropriate patient-specific data can be retrieved only by those who have legitimate access to it. HDOs are also seen to collect valid and reliable data so that quality of health care can be tracked and public policy can be promulgated. This vision includes the building of computerized patient records that can be shared by providers of care while still maintaining patient confidentiality.

Generalist Practitioners Are Beginning To Manage Specialists

This is already beginning to happen in MCOs. The doctor is no longer a "sage on the stage"instead, he is a "guide on the side." Staff or group model HMOs are hiring NPPCPs (nonphysician primary care practitioners), such as nurse practitioners and physician's assistants, who follow treatment algorithms and refer only a small percentage of patients on to a doctor. More and more, generalist health practitioners (such as nurse practitioners and case managers) will be cuing single-discipline practitioners (such as medical specialists) on what the patient needs and how the treatment plan should be structured.

Chronic care service often involves the heavy use of nonmedical interventions. Case managers in certain settings are now providing contracting with others or directing service providers who are doing telephone triage, case management, or alternative and ancillary health services.

The Demedicalization of Health Care Is Occurring in Our Lifetime

The process of care is beginning to be negotiated, rather than professionally dominated. Nurses, now the linchpin of the system, are taking over the gatekeeper role that physicians have held in some MCOs. The implication of a managed-care health system is an oversupply of physicians and relegation of specialty providers to a technical status. As the population ages and it is becoming evident to the mainstream that there is no cure for chronic disease, a change in consciousness about what constitutes health and medical care is sparking interest in alternative therapies.

Most people, including high-risk "communities of solution" (e.g., children, the elderly, certain occupational or employee groups), do quite nicely without allopathic interventions most of the time. As the point of service moves out of the hospital to the home and over the telephone and computer, people will regain control over their bodies and their health. The goal of the case manager is for every patient to begin to practice at being his or her own case manager.

The Focus on Curing Is Shifting to a Focus on Caring

Now that most people are living longer, and living with chronic diseases, more value is being placed on the (traditionally women's) work of caring. This will have multiple ramifications concerning the ethics of how resources are allocated and what care is considered appropriate. By doing away with the myth of the cure, human beings can focus on their individual life mission. This mission involves the challenges of disease and disability that each person must face while participating in a life quest for wholeness, a healing journey.

The Focus on Physical Health Is Shifting to a Focus on Spiritual Health

The widespread rethinking of the value of technologic interventions to cure the body will continue, with more focus on what the patient brings to the health process. A person's comfort and control of his or her inner environment are as important to health as his or her external environment. Scientists involved in the fields of psychoneuroimmunology[4] and brain-mind research[5] have concluded that there are grounds for believing in the existence of a nonmaterial basis for how human beings think and feel. Thus, the spiritual self controls the brain and the brain controls the body. Health care professionals, including case managers, need to have a level of comfort with this concept and its possible effects on the case manager role and treatment plans.

THE FUTURE OF HEALTH SERVICE REIMBURSEMENT

Now that the fee-for-service system is waning, it is time to review the ways that health services have been reimbursed and what the future holds.

Insurance-based health care risk exposure techniques have evolved in three stages.

In Stage 1, costs were controlled by benefit design and retrospective utilization review. Case management had a stopgap role in cost containment. Insurance payers excluded benefits payments where they could and used case management only to stretch benefits dollars when they were faced with high exposure to expenses related to a catastrophic case.

Stage 2 was characterized by utilization management through capitation and clinical algorithms (critical paths or CareMAPs)—the "care management" described in Chapter 7. The focus was still on more efficient utilization, which did not necessarily make the patient's *care* any more efficient or effective since critical pathing is process centered rather than patient centered.

Stage 3, which is beginning now, involves moderating the use of medical resources by managing demand and by optimizing outcomes through use of health status assessments and behavioral health interventions. Such strategies exemplify true case management, which improves the efficiency and effectiveness of care by being patient centered.

Demand Management

We have already mentioned what is being done with telephone help lines to reduce the demand for health services (see Chapter 2). Better educated and information-seeking consumers will be able to use their personal computer and CD-ROM data discs to find the answers to many of their health-related questions and even to visualize parts of the human anatomy. MCOs are now using telephone help lines to encourage this phenomenon further.

People tend not to seek medical services if they can answer questions concerning their personal health without having to seek care. Thus, demand for services declines as the perception of the need for services declines. Some studies suggest that as much as 25 to 50 percent of the variation in the use of care is determined by the perception of need.[6]

Health Status Assessment and Behavioral Health Interventions

In Stage 3, managed-care entities and HMOs will increasingly be using health status measures such as the Health Status Questionnaire (HSQ) and TyPE specifications to trigger case management and evaluate the effectiveness of interventions.

As discussed in Chapter 6, such psychometric instruments have shown superior validity in measuring health outcomes compared to the usual biometric measures that physicians have provided. Because health is a multidimensional biopsychosocial phenomenon whose locus of control resides within the individual, the evaluation of the appropriateness and effectiveness of the interventions needs to be patient centered.

Aside from economic status, the factors that have been shown to lead to poor health and functioning tend to be perceptual, attitudinal, and related to social support and lifestyle issues. The HSQ and TyPE instruments can provide a preintervention snapshot of the patient's self-rated health and well-being. They can also provide a clinical database of diagnostic categories (such as angina or diabetes).

The acute care medical model has been unable to provide appropriate interventions for the complex biopsychosocial phenomenon that is health. The services offered by MCOs could be more efficient and effective if behavioral health interventions were offered as part of the repertoire of services. Those patients who rate their health poorly are the ones who should be case managed, and those case managers should have the training and information support to guide patients to stay on the agreed-upon treatment paths. This would make case management much more effective in terms of traditional return-on-investment measures and would provide a service that could speak to the real needs of the 10 to 20 percent of patients who account for 80 to 90 percent of the utilization.

The following are some advantages to using HSQs and behavioral health interventions in a comprehensive health management program:

1. enhanced treatment choices for subscribers and primary care physicians
2. interventions that are low cost compared to conventional medical treatments
3. decreased exposure by plans and providers to lawsuits through improved communication and decreased numbers of invasive procedures
4. improved physical and emotional functioning on the part of participating subscribers
5. information to improve goal setting for patients faced with chronic disease
6. improved compliance of participating patients with their plan of care
7. responsiveness of the managed-care plan to new techniques of health interventions that specifically address chronic disease

NEW DIRECTIONS IN BEHAVIORAL HEALTH

Theory and Implications for Practice: Stress

The foundation of behavioral health is the ability to cope with the stress of life. Case managers, in the present and in the future, need to be well grounded in stress theory so that they can find appropriate types of interventions to offer to patients and families.

Stress is generally taken to be indicated by physiological components that can be quantifiably measured and psychological components, such as feeling states, that are subjectively reported.[7]

Hans Selye is generally acknowledged to have demonstrated the link between stress and illness.[8] Later he developed a theory of the general adaptation syndrome (GAS), characterized by a period of *alarm*, then *resistance*, and finally *exhaustion* as reactions to stress.[9] This construct is still useful in understanding the reactions of patients and their families to disease, as the letdown of energy and motivation often occurs after the crisis period has passed. Selye later amended his view to postulate that stress could promote a positive influence. He used the term *heterostasis* to refer to the body's proactive mechanism to maintain a heightened level of resistance or be energized by stress.

But what is stress? Antonovsky defined a *stressor* as a demand that taxes or exceeds the resources of a system, *tension* as the response to the stressor, and *stress* itself as the reaction when one has failed to reduce the tension. He believed that a person needs a sense of confidence or *coherence*—a sense that his or her internal and external environments will be predictable and manageable.[10] This model makes sense when we look at the phenomenon of hypertension. This "silent killer" plays a significant role in the first and third causes of death in the United States, heart disease and stroke.[11] Hypertension is the result of stress when one is unable to reduce the effect of stressors on one's daily life. Hypertension is a maladaptive coping mechanism predisposed by heredity and reinforced by learning. While hypertension may block the subjective feeling of stress, it does not block its long-term effect on health.

More recently, Antonovsky put forth a theory of what he called *salutogenesis*. Again, the central idea is coherence. If individuals appraise their world as comprehensible, manageable, and meaningful, they will be more able to cope with the stressors they encounter in their daily lives. Antonovsky sketched out five stages of the "salutogenic effect":

1. The individual sees him- or herself as linked to others in the world rather than isolated.

2. The individual is able to make sense of the stimuli to which he or she is subjected. The stimuli are perceived as information rather than "noise."
3. The individual develops internal processes to sort, translate, code, and integrate information so that it can be used successfully to manage his or her environment.
4. There are resources available in the environment to translate plans into behavior. These resources include motivational, emotional, and cognitive resources.
5. The individual appraises the feedback that he or she obtains from interactions with the environment as helpful information rather than as a sign of rejection by others.[12]

The case manager's role in stress management is to facilitate the salutogenic effect by recognizing the patient's and family's relative ability to appraise their situation effectively, and by involving them in positive actions that can give a sense of coherence to the activities that handle the stress of the disease/illness process. During the interview process, the "self-talk" that patients use to describe their illness experience can be used to assess patients' effectiveness in coping with the major life crisis that the illness experience engenders.

Many chronic illnesses place more demands on patients and their families than they can bear alone. Perhaps this is why so many older spouses die within a year of their mate's passing. It is very useful for the case manager to explore what kinds of support groups are available.

The inability of people to respond to the stress of life tends to drive up the costs of medical care because medical care is provided to address complaints of physical pain rather than their emotional origin. Case managers should be aware of the predisposition by some patients to engender inappropriate medical treatments with their somatization of psychic pain.

Psychoneuroimmunology

The field of psychoneuroimmunology (PNI) explores how the brain and central nervous system, the endocrine system, and the immune system act as one functioning system. Previously, it was believed that the brain communicated by electrical conduction of nerve impulses, but this model did not satisfactorily answer issues concerning feeling states and the body's reaction to disease as mediated by the mind. In the early 1980s Candice Pert discovered that the neuropeptide endorphin was manufactured by the brain to produce a natural painkilling drug. This drug was bound to receptors in the brain and other areas of the body that configured themselves to require the drug given the body's reaction to pain and other phenomena. Now a number of neuropeptides have been identified, and disturbances in their balance have been linked to mood states and behavioral maladaptations. For example, serotonin reuptake inhibitor drugs (such as Prozac) have been shown to alter a person's ability to perceive stressful events and to enable the person to cope better. The uptake of serotonin, a neuropeptide, causes some individuals to appraise their environment in such a way that they are not able to cope with stress in a successfully adaptive manner.

Pert suggested that the bidirectional network of neuropeptides and their receptors is the physiologic basis for the body's flow of energy and the material basis for emotions.[13] More recently, Sir John Eccles postulated that the self controls the brain by selective attention and a lifetime of learning.[14] That is to say, the intentionality of each individual makes the brain work. The brain, in turn, makes the body work. This means we each have a say in our own destiny in terms of our ability to cope with the impairment of physiology due to disease. It also suggests the existence of a nonmaterial being (a spirit or soul) that controls the body.

Such research challenges us to redefine health in a way that takes into account the powerful influences of thought and emotion on the body, and in a way that makes sense to each patient and family that the case manager encounters.

Treatments

Disease and Pain Management

Behavioral health treatments for identified disease states and for disease- or injury-related chronic pain have been refined over a number of years to include a repertoire of strategies. Social support is increasingly being recognized as a crucial component of treatment. Support groups range from self-help groups that share information and treatment modalities concerning single diseases or injuries, such as head or spinal cord injuries, to highly structured "therapeutic communities" that assist patients to cope with cancer or other life-threatening diseases that involve long periods of treatment and exact a toll on the coping resources of the patient and family.

One of the best known success stories concerning the positive effect of social support on treatment outcomes comes from David Spiegel's work with cancer patients. His book *Living beyond Limits* outlined his philosophy that cancer treatment should aim for a midpoint between the materialistic view of the patient as a helpless victim of cancer and the disembodied spiritualism of Simonton and others who seek to fix the problem in the mind to make it disappear from the body.[15] Spiegel's approach attempts to make the most of patients' personal and social resources in the service of living a full life by assisting them to face realistically the limits imposed by life and illness. Spiegel is known for having remarkably improved survival rates for breast cancer patients which incorporated his regimen of social support. Patients are urged to "take charge" of their therapy in order to have a better quality of life and hopefully live beyond the limits of their diagnosis.

Speigel outlined five criteria for successful support groups:

1. patients with similar medical problems
2. excellent group leadership (i.e., at least a licensed professional)
3. a comfortable setting for meetings
4. reasonable rate of payment for the service
5. a supportive atmosphere in the group

Certain types of people seem to find support groups more appealing than others. Women and those with more education, an existing orientation toward self-care, or prior experience in psychotherapy seem to seek out and remain in self-help support groups.[16]

Many support groups incorporate various forms of instruction—not only the goal-setting techniques described in Chapter 10, but also strategies that specifically address the identified disorder. For example, Dean Ornish's programs for cardiac patients gather patients in weekly support groups in which they are introduced to stress reduction or relaxation techniques, a very low-fat (less than 10 percent of calories from fat) diet, a regimen of moderate exercise, and medical supervision. The weekly support group meetings give the patients a chance to compare their strategies and progress with others who are encountering similar issues. Ornish's experimental group showed significant reduction in the occlusions of coronary arteries, whereas his control group of similar patients with coronary artery disease showed advances in their blockages. Both groups were measured before and after the interventions by cardiac catheterization.[17]

Jon Kabat-Zinn's programs for patients who suffer from intractable and chronic pain, or who in other ways are not responding to their treatment regimens, teach *mindfulness meditation*, the systematic cultivation of mindfulness. *Mindfulness* is the state of resting in the moment and paying attention to one's mind and body without trying to change or control anything. Techniques include *sitting meditation*, in which one follows one's breath; a *body scan*, in which one systematically concentrates one's awareness on the various regions of the body recognizing sensations and emotions and letting them go; *yoga*, in which one goes through the postures slowly and with full awareness, exploring and working near the body's limits; *walking meditation*, in which one devotes one's attention entirely to the experience of walking; and experiments in applying mindfulness to any other activity of daily life.[18]

Mindfulness practice reduces stress, promotes relaxation, and strengthens the individual's coping powers. Further, and paradoxically, tuning into physical and psychic pain and observing its fluctuations is a more effective way of reducing it than the tactics of ignoring it or distracting oneself. Also, mindfulness techniques prove particularly helpful for patients who must be sensitive to their physical limitation (such as low back pain), yet who need to remain active and wish to extend the limits of their ability.

Drug and Alcohol Treatment

The best known self-help groups are Alcoholics Anonymous and other twelve-step programs. The 12 steps are:

1. Admit powerlessness over substance abuse.
2. Believe that a higher power can restore one to sanity.
3. Turn life and will over to God.
4. Take a moral inventory of self.
5. Admit to self and other the exact nature of one's wrongs.
6. Be ready to have God remove one's character deficits.
7. Ask God to remove the deficits.
8. Make a list of persons harmed and resolve willingness to make amends.
9. Make direct amends where possible.
10. Continue to take personal inventory.
11. Improve conscious contact with God through prayer and meditation.
12. Carry the message of spiritual awakening to others; practice these principles in all affairs.[19]

The 12-step approach is widely copied, and many drug and alcohol programs refer patients to a 12-step program as part of their routine therapeutic regimen. However, the efficacy of drug and alcohol treatment programs (apart from AA and NA programs, which are free) is in question, and many behavioral managed-care programs no longer pay for services as they once did because the recidivism rate is so high. Drug and alcohol treatments are being widely rethought, and programs are being retooled.

Case management in this area, though it may benefit from some of the tools mentioned here, is beyond the scope of this book.

Medical Offset Programs

Medical offset research is a type of outcomes research developed by Cummings and others at the Kaiser-Permanente Health Plan in California to discover ways to offset the costs of the 60 percent of primary care visits due to somaticized stress rather than physical disease.[20] Kaiser developed a program to identify 68 psychological/psychiatric conditions so that 68 focused interventions could be devised. These programs use brief, intermittent psychotherapy to solve immediate problems and give the patient a greater repertoire of responses to stress.

By involving patients in brief individual therapy, group therapy, psychoeducational sessions, and (for a small subset of patients) therapy spaced over intervals of several months, Kaiser was able to show a return on investment of almost $9 on medical expenses not spent for every $1 spent on psychological services.

Among the interventions used in medical offset programs, *brief therapy* has come to mean therapy that uses cognitive and problem-solving modalities. The therapy generally lasts from three to eight visits, and its effectiveness generally depends on whether the therapist can provide a mode of intervention that matches the patient's style and needs. *Time-effective therapy* refers to therapy that assumes that certain patients will have crisis periods throughout their life requiring therapy. It includes drug regimens as well as spaced psychotherapy, and utilizes interventions that attempt to take individual patient needs and diagnosis into account.

SUMMARY

A variety of new behavioral health interventions, based on new research exploring the crucial role of patients' attitudes, beliefs, and behaviors in determining health outcomes, are changing the face of health care. Case managers who can use this information to improve patients' health by identifying coping issues and making a broad range of medical and not-so-traditional options available to them will engage patients in a process that will enhance the future of all.

NOTES

1. J. Flower, The *Other* Revolution in Health Care, *Wired* (Jan. 1994):108–113.
2. R. Allison, Demystifying CHIN Technologies, *Journal of the Community Medical Network Society* 1, no. 1 (1995):24–27.

3. M.S. Donaldson and K.N. Lohr, eds., *Health Data in the Information Age: Use, Disclosure and Privacy* (Washington, D.C.: National Academy Press, 1994), 17.

4. C. Pert et al., Neuropeptides and Their Receptors: A Psychosomatic Network, *Journal of Immunology* 135 (1986):820S–826S.

5. J.C. Eccles, *How the SELF Controls Its BRAIN* (New York: Springer-Verlag, 1994).

6. C. Russell, *What Determines Demand?* (Golden, Colo.: Health Decisions, Inc., 1994).

7. L.A. Bieliauskas, *Stress and Its Relationship to Health and Illness* (Boulder, Colo.: Westview Press, 1982).

8. H. Selye, A Sydrome Produced by Diverse Nocuous Agents, *Nature* 138 (1936):32.

9. H. Selye, *Stress without Distress* (New York: J.B. Lippincott Co., 1974).

10. A. Antonovsky, *Health, Stress and Coping* (San Francisco: Jossey-Bass, Inc., Publishers, 1979).

11. J.B. McKinlay and S.M. McKinlay, A Review of the Evidence Concerning the Impact of Medical Interventions on Recent Mortality and Morbidity in the United States, *International Journal of Health Services* 19 (1989):181–208.

12. A. Antonovsky, A Sociological Critique of the "Well-Being Movement," *Advances: The Journal of Mind-Body Health* 10, no. 3 (1994):6–11.

13. C. Pert, The Material Basis for Emotions, *Whole Earth Review* (1988):106–111.

14. Eccles, *How the SELF.*

15. D. Spiegel, *Living beyond Limits* (New York: Times Books, 1993).

16. C.E. Sutherland and M.S. Goldstein, Joining a Healing Community for Cancer: Who and Why? *Social Science in Medicine* 35 (1992):323–333.

17. D. Ornish et al., Can Lifestyle Changes Reverse Coronary Heart Disease? *Lancet* 336 (1990):129–133.

18. J. Kabat-Zinn, *Full Catastrophe Living* (New York: Delacorte Press, 1990).

19. Alcoholics Anonymous World Services, *Twelve Steps and Twelve Traditions* (New York: 1952).

20. N.A. Cummings, The Successful Application of Medical Offset in Program Planning and in Clinical Delivery, *Managed Care Quarterly* 2, no. 2 (1994): 1–6.

Appendix A

Forms and Tools

The forms and tools contained in this appendix are typical of those used by independent case management companies. The initial evaluation tool takes issues into account that most nursing assessments do not cover, such as the mechanism of injury, education, employment history, rehabilitation obstacles and facilitators, and cost projections. The initial evaluation tool is compressed here to save space, but should be expanded to about five to six pages or templated on a computer file if the case manager uses a laptop. If the latter is the case, time can be saved because the information does not have to be rewritten for the subsequent report.

REHABILITATION CASE MANAGEMENT INITIAL EVALUATION TOOL

TO: _____   Claimant: _____
FROM: _____   File # _____
Date of report _____   Date of Loss (DOL) _____
Social Security Number _____

Diagnosis/disability list, with ICD-9 code:
1.
2.
3.

Introduction/summary statement:

Profile:
Name: Age:
Date of birth: Significant other:
Ht/Wt: Date of encounter:
Right or left hand dominant:

Brief history of accident:

Hospitalizations: (aftermath of accident; when, where, why of all other hospitalizations)

Surgeries:

Medication/indications:

Drug allergies, drug usage if known:

Current Treatment:

Physicians: (List in order of importance; specify address, phone/fax, and other board specialty.)

Physical/functional problems related to the accident: (list)

Cognitive problems: (loss of consciousness?)

Past medical history: (surgeries, hospitalizations, medication)

continues

Initial Evaluation Tool (continued)

Family/social history: (Detail home environment, describe house and barriers if applicable, describe family structure and support, type of employment of household members.)

Education/employment history: (Important for documenting lost work time, physical work that may prevent claimant from returning to same work. Calculate lost time from work/lost wages/RTW date if requested.)

Rehabilitation facilitators: (motivation, supportive family, doctor's view, prognosis)

Rehabilitation obstacles: (list)

Assessment: (Case manager's assessment of the above information and general prediction of care needs and events. Should include expected outcome, including measures needed to determine the effectiveness of the treatments.)

Cost/utilization projections: (medical and other cost category needs, project involvement of case management)

Recommendations: (list of what actions should be taken by whom)

CONSENT FOR THE RELEASE OF MEDICAL INFORMATION

I, _____ , hereby consent to the

release of medical information to _____ . I authorize

all providers of care to me to release any records of my care to these individuals.

Signed:_____

Date: _____

INDEPENDENT MEDICAL EXAMINATION

Claimant Letter

RE:
FILE NO:
INSURED:
DOL:

Dear _____ :

_____ Company has requested that we arrange an
Independent Medical Exam for you. I have scheduled you to see:

      Physician: Type of Dr.:

      Address:

      Phone:

      Date & Time:

Please note that your attorney has also been notified of this appointment [omit if no attorney]. It has been scheduled far enough in advance in order for you or your attorney to contact me should there be any questions or concerns regarding the appointment.

Please take any x-rays and medical records you have to this appointment. Should you have the need to cancel, please call the physician's office or our office at least 48 hours before your scheduled appointment. A no-show or late cancellation fee of $_____ will be charged by this physician.

Please give me a call if you have any questions.

Cert. #

INDEPENDENT MEDICAL EXAMINATION

Doctor Letter

RE:
FILE NO:
INSURED:
DOL:

Dear _____ :

Thank you for consenting to see the above-named patient for an Independent Medical Exam on _____.

The following information is pertinent:

In your report I would appreciate your addressing the following:

1. What is your diagnosis?
2. Is this condition solely a result of this accident?
3. Has this patient reached maximum medical improvement? If not, can you project when this should occur?
4. Any other comments regarding the current medical status.

Please forward your bill to:

ATTENTION: (Adjuster)

PLEASE FORWARD YOUR REPORT TO ME AT THE ABOVE ADDRESS WITHIN TEN (10) DAYS AFTER THE EXAMINATION. I have enclosed a return envelope for your convenience.

It is my understanding that your fee for this IME is $ _____ ; $ _____ no-show fee. No continued treatment is authorized.

JOB DESCRIPTION: TO BE FILLED OUT BY CASE MANAGER AS PART OF AN EFFORT TO PLACE A PREVIOUSLY INJURED WORKER

Date: _____

Company: _____   Employer Contact Person: _____

Address: _____   Phone Number: _____

_____

Job Title: _____   Wages: _____ /hr. _____ /wk.

Hours Worked: Per Day _____   Per Week _____ Breaks _____

Jobs Duties/Responsibilities:

Physical Capacity: Please complete all categories

Standing (Hours) _____	How Often ____	Lifting (Pounds) ____	How Often _____
Sitting (Hours) _____	How Often ____	Driving in Auto _____	How Often _____
Walking (Hours) _____	How Often ____	Climbing _____	How Often _____
Bending _____	How Often ____	Reaching _____	How Often _____
Push/Pull w/Arms ____	How Often ____	Stooping _____	How Often _____
Push/Pull w/Legs ____	How Often ____	Squatting _____	How Often _____
Push/Pull w/Body ____	How Often ____		

Equipment/Machines Operated:

Physical Environment:

Special Consideration/Job Modification (if any):

EMPLOYER CONTACT Personal Visit: _____   Phone Contact: _____

Position Currently Available: Yes ____   No: _____

Accepting Application: Yes _____   No _____   Submitted: Yes ____ No ____

Interview Scheduled: Yes _____   No _____   Date: _____

Job Offered: Yes _____   No _____   Date: _____

Applicant Accepted _____   Refused _____

Employer Comments:

Employer Signature: _____   Date: _____

PHYSICIAN VERIFICATION

I have reviewed the above job description of employment for _____ and feel that this job is within his/her physical abilities of performing.

PHYSICIAN COMMENTS:

Physician Signature: _____   Date: _____

CASE MANAGER COMMENTS:

Case Manager: _____   Date: _____

PROSPECTIVE UTILIZATION REVIEW DATA SHEET FOR AMBULATORY ENCOUNTERS

Date _____

Patient _____ SS# _____

Address _____

Date of birth _____ Sex _____

Insurer _____

Claim # _____ Date of injury _____

Employer _____

Diagnosis _____ ICD-9 code(s) _____

— —

Provider _____

Provider contact person (to provide additional clinical information) _____

Address _____

Phone _____ Fax _____

Degrees/certifications _____

Tax ID# _____ Projected dates of service _____

Projected # visits _____ Projected stop date _____

Treatment goals _____

Treatment modalities _____

_____

Expected functional/health outcomes _____

_____

INSTRUCTIONS FOR CASE MANAGER CONTACT SHEET

The Nurse Case Manager Daily Contact Sheet and the code list that accompanies it are a tool to track the productivity of case managers. This tool was developed for a nursing home, but is based on a format that is common with external insurance case managers. It can be adapted to other settings.

The contact sheet lists all those residents or patients with whom the case manager has interacted in an official capacity, describes briefly what activity was performed, and states who else was involved, and how much time was spent. (The expectation is for a documented six hours of productive time per day. This figure comes from experience with external rehabilitation case managers.) The case managers were given these sheets after they were trained as a group and had acclimated to the role. No expectation was given to them initially regarding documenting their productive time.

Initially wide variation was found in the documented productive time of the case managers. After feedback stating when to fill the sheets out and telling case managers that their time was expected to be productive, the case managers themselves shared techniques for remembering to track their time and being more focused in their activities. After three months, a report was prepared showing the productive time of all the case managers in graph form, but without identifying individuals.The results were shared with the case managers, and a discussion ensued as to ways to be more time-effective. The standard of 6.4 hours of productive contact time was initiated after the learning period passed, and this expectation was added to the job description.

**NURSE CASE MANAGER
DAILY CONTACT SHEET**

Case Manager: Date:

Resident	Room	Description of Services	Activity	Contact	Time

NURSE CASE MANAGER
CONTACT SHEET CODES

Activity Codes

A1 Initial resident contact; includes physical assessment
A2 Chart review; includes data gathering for any documentation purpose
A3 Clinical review; includes all issues relating to clinical problems
A4 Follow-up contact and correspondence
A5 Review correspondence
A6 Telephone to
A7 Telephone from
A8 Planning meeting
A9 Coordinate care; includes making appointments, directing other caregivers, etc.
A10 Coordinate admission/discharge

Contact Codes

C1 Resident/client
C2 Family/POA
C3 Doctor
C4 Social service
C5 Clergy
C6 Physical therapy
C7 Other therapists
C8 Consultant
C9 Dietary
C10 Activities
C11 Other in-house nursing staff
C12 Other (note who in description column)

Appendix B

Glossary

꧁꧂

This glossary of terms is designed to support a wide variety of case management activity. Legal, insurance, vocational, utilization review, and some clinical terms applying to high-risk or traumatically injured groups are included. Also included are terms that would support an improved understanding of health measurement and quality improvement activities.

Absolute Risk. Quantitative difference in the risk of disease or death among an exposed population and the risk among the unexposed. Difference between the incidence rate in an exposed population and the incidence rate in the unexposed one.

Accelerated-compensation event (ACE). A class of medically caused injuries determined by experts to be normally avoidable if patients are given good care.

Source: The glossary includes terms adapted or reprinted from *Home Care: An Emerging Solution to the Nation's Health Care Crisis*, with permission of Olsten Kimberly QualityCare, © 1993; *CCM Certification Guide*, with permission of the Foundation for Rehabilitation Certification, Education and Research, © 1993; *Health Insurance Answer Book: 1994 Cumulative Supplement* by Thomas A. Darold, with permission of Panel Publishers, a division of Aspen Publishers, Inc., 36 West 44th Street, Suite 1316, New York, NY 10036, © 1994; and *Case Management Practice*, with permission of the Foundation for Rehabilitation Certification, Education and Research, © 1993.

Proposed as an alternative standard of liability for medical malpractice. A patient would receive compensation if an ACE occurred, without determining whether fault or negligence was involved in that particular case.

Access/accessibility of care. The ease with which patients obtain the care they need when they need it; a component of quality of care.

Activities of daily living (ADLs). Activities in the nonoccupational environment arising from daily living needs (e.g., mobility, personal hygiene, dressing, sleeping, eating, and skills required for community living).

Acute care hospital. A hospital or component of a hospital that provides care for acute and chronic medical, surgical, obstetrical, and intensive care patients.

Acute Physiology, Age, and Chronic Health Evaluation (APACHE) System. The system developed by Apache Medical System, Inc., to provide risk-adjusted predicted mortality and length-of-stay outcomes for critical care patients.

Adjusted average per capita cost (AAPCC). An estimate of the average per capita cost incurred by Medicare per beneficiary in the fee-for-service system, adjusted by county for differences in age, sex, disability status, Medicaid eligibility, and institutional status.

Adjuster. A ratio figure that alters relative values to calibrate payment more accurately to a defined population, such as Medicare beneficiaries. Also, a claims representative for an insurance company who functions to investigate claims for damage, estimates the costs to settle claims, and authorizes payment for services necessary to settle claims.

Agency. A relationship between two parties in which the first party authorizes the second to act as agent on behalf of the first, or a contractual arrangement between two parties managed by a third party, an agent.

Agency for Health Care Policy and Research. Component of U.S. Public Health Service charged with medical effectiveness research and facilitating the development of clinical practice guidelines.

Agent. A party authorized to act on behalf of another and to give the other an account of such actions.

Algorithm. An explicit description of an ordered sequence of steps to be taken in patient care under specified circumstances.

Ancillary services. Traditionally, hospital services that are adjuncts to the diagnosis and treatment of patient's conditions, including laboratory medicine and pathology, diagnostic and therapeutic radiology, and physical and occupational therapy.

Appeal. The process whereby a court of appeals reviews the record of written materials from a court proceeding to determine if errors were made that might lead to a reversal of the trial court's decision, or a formal request to reconsider a determination not to certify an admission, extension of stay, or other health care service.

Appropriateness of care. The degree to which the correct care is provided, given current state-of-the-art knowledge; a component of quality of care.

Approved charge. The amount Medicare pays a physician based on the Medicare Fee Schedule or its transition rules. Physicians may bill beneficiaries for an additional amount, subject to the limiting charge.

Assignment (Medicare). A beneficiary's directive to Medicare to pay benefits directly to the physician or supplier. Medicare will do this only if the physician accepts Medicare's allowed charge as payment in full (guarantees not to balance bill). (See **balance billing, nonparticipating physician, participating physician,** and **supplier program.**)

Assistant at surgery. An individual who has the necessary qualifications to participate in a particular operation and actively assists in performing the surgery. Medicare will pay for the service only when performed by a physician or a physician assistant.

Assumption of risk. A doctrine based on voluntary exposure to a known risk. It is distinguished from contributory negligence (which is based on carelessness) in that it involves the comprehension that a peril is to be encountered as well as the willingness to encounter it.

Attending physician. The physician with primary responsibility for the care provided to a patient in a hospital or other health care facility.

Authorization to pay benefits. A provision in a medical claim form by which the insured directs the insurance company to pay any benefits directly to the provider of care on whose charges the claim is based.

Automatic reinsurance. A type of reinsurance in which the insurer must cede and the reinsuring company must accept all risks within certain contractually defined areas (also called **treaty reinsurance**). The reinsuring company undertakes in advance to grant reinsurance to the extent specified in the agreement in every case in which the ceding company accepts the application and retains its own limit.

Balance billing. A physician charge exceeding an approved payment lock or fee schedule.

Beneficiary. A person eligible for benefits under an insurance plan. Under Part B of Medicare, Americans over 65, many disabled individuals, and certain individuals with end-stage renal disease can become beneficiaries by paying a monthly premium.

Benefits. The amount payable by an insurance company to the claimant, assignee, or beneficiary under a specific coverage.

Bias. A preconceived personal preference or inclination that influences the way in which a measurement, analysis, assessment, or procedure is performed or reported; a systematic error in measurement.

Bill audit. The review of hospital, physician, durable medical equipment, and health care service provider bills for inaccuracies or overbilling.

Binary variables. Variables that have two possible outcomes (e.g., dead or alive, male or female; also referred to as **dichotomous variables**).

Biological variation. Patient health-related factors (beyond the control of providers) that influence the outcome of care.

Bundling. The use of a single payment for a group of related services. For an example of bundling, see **global surgery policy**.

Business alliances. Groups of business companies allied to reduce health care costs by jointly purchasing medical services.

Capitation. A method of payment for health services in which the health care provider is paid a fixed amount for each person over a specific amount of time regardless of the actual number or nature of services provided to each person.

Caregiver. A family member, volunteer, or medical professional charged with providing care in the home setting.

CareMAP. Cause-and-effect grid that identifies patient/family and staff behaviors against a time line by case type. The MAPs (multidisciplinary action plans) are nonconceptual and visual and contain common clinical language. The four parts are (1) *time line:* per diagnosis and projected resource use projections; (2) *index of problems:* list, with intermediate expectations and behavioral outcome criteria; (3) *critical path:* consensus statement as to treatment process and progression; and (4) *variance record:* patient focused, but data analyzed for population variables. The term **CareMAP** comes from work done by the Center for Case Management in Natick, Massachusetts.

Carrier. An insurance company or administrator of benefits under an insurance contract.

Case-based review. Approach to quality-of-care evaluation based on review of individual medical records by health professionals who make judgments as to whether the care delivered was of acceptable quality.

Case-control study. A study that involves the identification of persons with the disease or condition of interest (cases) and similar group of persons without the disease or condition of interest (controls). Cases and controls are compared with respect to some existing or past attribute or exposure believed to be causally related to the disease or condition. Also referred to as a **retrospective study** because this research approach proceeds from effect to cause.

Case mix. The relative frequency of different diagnoses or conditions among patients at a facility. Case-mix adjustment is used to separate the effects of the care given from those of preexisting health status and other factors (such as age and socioeconomic status) that affect outcome measures.

Case reserve. The dollar amount stated in a claims file that represents an estimate of the amount still unpaid.

Case series. A study that reports on a consecutive collection of patients treated in a similar manner without a concurrent control group.

Certification. A determination by a utilization review organization that an admission, extension of stay, or other health care service has been reviewed and that on the basis of the information provided, it meets the medical review requirements of the applicable health benefit plan.

Charge. Statement of purpose given to a group of experts convened to develop a set of function-specific indicators during the indicator developmental process.

Chronic. Describes condition or disease of long duration showing little change; opposite of **acute**.

Claim. A request for payment of reparation for a loss covered by an insurance contract.

Claimant. The person filing the claim to whom benefits are to be paid by the claims administrator.

Claims administrator. Any entity that reviews and determines whether to pay claims to enrollees, physicians, hospitals, or others on behalf of the health benefit plan. Such payment determinations are made on the basis of contract provisions. Claims administrators may be insurance companies, self-insured employers, third-party administrators, or other private contractors.

Claims cost control. Efforts made by an insurer both inside and outside its own organization to restrain and direct claims payments so that health insurance premium dollars are used as efficiently as possible.

Claims data. Data derived from providers' claims to third-party payers.

Claims-made policy. A professional liability insurance policy that covers the holder for a period in which a claim of malpractice is made. The alleged act of malpractice may have occurred at some previous time, but the policy insures the holder when the claim is made.

Claims reserves. Funds reserved by an insurer to settle incurred but unpaid claims; may also include reserves for potential claims fluctuation.

Claims service representative. A person who investigates losses and settles claims for an insurance carrier or the insured. **Adjuster** is a synonymous, although less preferred, term.

Clinical criteria. The written policies, decision rules, medical protocols, or guides used by a utilization review organization to determine certification.

Clinical device. A defined hospital service (e.g., obstetrics, general medicine, cardiology, oncology).

Clinical experience. Expertise gained through professional clinical practice (e.g., any combination of direct patient care in a specialty area, home health, or general clinical area for which the applicant is licensed or certified).

Clinical outcomes. Information about the results of patient diagnosis and treatment (e.g., mortality, length of stay).

Clinical prediction rule. A rule for interpreting clinical data to predict a clinical event.

Clinical quality. The quality of care as measured by outcome measurement data.

Clinical target. A clinical sign, symptom, or physiologic parameter that responds to medical treatment and is highly correlated with achieving the ultimate patient outcome intended by a practice guideline.

Code creep. The practice by health providers or billing offices of ICD-9 or CPT coding and billing for a greater intensity of service than was actually delivered.

Coding. A mechanism for identifying and defining physicians' services. Refers to Current Procedural Terminology (CPT) book, which lists service codes and their descriptions.

Cohort. A group of people defined by a common characteristic or set of characteristics.

Coinsurance. The percentage of balance of covered medical expenses that a beneficiary must pay after payment of the deductible. Under Medicare Part B, the beneficiary pays coinsurance of 20 percent of allowed charges.

Comorbidity. Coexisting, usually chronic conditions that may affect overall health and functional status beyond the effect(s) of the condition under consideration.

Compensation. An act that a court orders done (including money that a court or other tribunal orders to be paid) by a person whose acts or omissions have caused loss or injury in order to make the injured party "whole" with respect to the loss.

Complication. Condition that arises during a hospital stay or health encounter that intensifies the utilization of service or prolongs the length of stay.

Comprehensive major medical insurance. A form of major medical expense insurance (written with an initial deductible) that can substitute for separate policies providing basic hospital, surgical, and medical benefits.

Concurrent care. A circumstance in which nonconsultative services are rendered by more than one physician during a given period of time.

Concurrent insurance. Insurance of a person under two or more policies providing similar or identical coverages (usually avoided in group insurance).

Concurrent review. A form of utilization review that tracks the progress of a patient during treatment; conducted on site or by telephone.

Concurrent validity. The extent to which a measure correlates with other measures of the same theme. For example, do scores from a 5-item measure of pain correlate well with scores from a 25-item measure of pain?

Confidential communications. Certain classes of communications that the law will not permit to be divulged; in general, such communications pass between persons who stand in a confidential or fiduciary relationship to each other (or who, because of their relative situation, owe a special duty of secrecy and fidelity).

Construct validity. The extent to which the measurement fits in the conceptual framework of the quantity being measured; for example, whether physical function fits into the framework of what we think of as quality of life.

Contingency reserve. A reserve established to share among all policyholders the cost to the insurer of unpredictable catastrophic losses.

Continuity (or continuum) of care. The degree to which the care needed by the patient is coordinated among practitioners and across organizations and time; a component of quality of care.

Continuous quality improvement (CQI or QI). An approach to quality management that builds upon traditional quality assurance methods by emphasizing the organization and systems (rather than individuals), the need for customer definitions of quality, the need for objective data with which to analyze and improve processes, and the ideal that systems and performance can always improve even when high standards appear to have been met. Also called **total quality management** or TQM.

Conversion factor. The multiplicative factor applied to the relative value scale to produce a schedule of dollar amounts of payments for physicians.

Coordination of benefits (COB). A method of integrating benefits payable under more than one group health insurance plan so that the insured's benefits from all sources do not exceed 100 percent of his or her allowable medical expenses.

Copayment. Portion of a claim or medical expense that a claimant must pay out of pocket.

Cost. A measure of resource or value. Prices and charges may or may not reflect true resource consumption or public value. Direct costs are the costs required to produce a service, whereas indirect costs are all costs of an illness other than the direct costs.

Cost-based or cost-related reimbursement. A method of payment of medical care programs by third parties, typically Blue Cross plans or government agencies, for services delivered to patients.

Cost-benefit analysis. A form of economic assessment in which the costs of medical care are compared with the economic benefits of the care, with both costs and benefits expressed in units of currency; the benefits typically include reductions in future health care costs and increased earnings because of the improved health of those receiving the care.

Cost containment. The control of the overall cost of health care services within the health care delivery system. Costs are contained when the value of the resources committed to an activity is not considered to be excessive.

Cost-effectiveness. An economic evaluation in which alternative programs, services, or interventions are compared in terms of the cost per unit of clinical effect:

for example, cost per life saved, cost per millimeter of mercury of blood pressure lowering.

Cost sharing. The portion of payment for health expenses that the beneficiary must pay, including copayments (deductibles and coinsurance) and balance bills (see **balance billing, coinsurance, deductible**).

Cost shifting. A health care provider's compensation for the effect of decreased revenue from one payer by increasing charges to another payer.

Cost-utility analysis. A type of cost-effectiveness analysis in which outcomes are measured in terms of their social value. Cost is expressed per some incremental quality-of-life measure (e.g., cost per quality-adjusted life-year, cost per healthy days of life gained).

Coverage. (1) The aggregate of risks insured by a contract of insurance; (2) a major classification of benefits provided by a group policy (e.g., term life, weekly indemnity, major medical); (3) the amount of insurance or benefits stated in the group policy for which an insured is eligible.

Covered charges. Charges for medical care or supplies that, if incurred by an insured or other covered person, create a liability for the insurance under terms of a group policy.

Cross-examination. The questioning of a witness during a trial or deposition by the party opposing those who asked the person to testify.

Crosswalk. The assumed relationship between discontinued CPT codes and the new codes that replace them.

Current Procedural Terminology (CPT). The coding system for physicians' services developed by the American Medical Association; basis of the HCPCS coding system for physicians' services.

Customary charge. One of the screens previously used to determine the level for provider payment for a service under Medicare's customary, prevailing, and reasonable payment system. Customary charges were calculated as the physician's median charge for a given service over a prior 12-month period. (Also called **U&C charges.**)

Damages. Money awarded by the court to someone who has been injured (plaintiff) that must be paid by the party responsible for the injury (defendant). Normal damages are awarded when the injury is considered to be slight. Compensatory damages are awarded to repay or compensate the injured party for the loss that was incurred. Punitive damages are awarded when the injury is found to have been committed maliciously or in wanton disregard of the plaintiff's interests.

Data accuracy. The degree to which data required by indicators are free of mistakes (see **data quality**).

Database. An organized, comprehensive collection of data.

Data completeness. The degree to which data required by indicators exist and are available for use (see **data quality**).

Data element or data point. A single piece of information required by an indicator, subsequently aggregated with other data elements to identify indicator event occurrences.

Data pattern. An identifiable grouping of distribution of data characteristics that may trigger further investigation of the event monitored by an indicator.

Data quality. The degree to which data required by indicators are accurate and complete.

Data trend. The general direction of indicator rates over time that may trigger further investigation of the event monitored by an indicator.

Data verification process. Testing-phase process in which data required by indicators are verified for accuracy and completeness; process includes determination of why data quality may be suboptimal and how it may be improved.

Decision analysis. A systematic approach to decision making under conditions of uncertainty. It involves identifying all available choices and estimating the probabilities of potential outcomes for each in a series of decisions that have to be made regarding patient care. The analysis requires estimates of how patients value different health outcomes.

Deductible. A specified amount of covered medical expenses that a beneficiary must pay before receiving benefits. Medicare Part B has an annual deductible of $100.

Defendant. The person against whom an action is brought because of an alleged responsibility for violating one or more of the plaintiff's legally protected interests.

Dependent variable. Variable that takes on different values depending on the influence of other factors (e.g., age, sex).

Deposition. A sworn pretrial testimony given by a witness in response to oral and written questions and cross-examination. The deposition is transcribed and may be used for further pretrial investigation. It may also be presented at the trial if the witness cannot be present.

Desirable indicator. An outcome or process indicator that measures a desirable activity or result of care: for example, patient survival.

Diagnosis-related groups (DRGs). Groupings of patients by discharge diagnosis to measure a hospital's output. They are used for analysis and monitoring of the hospital's resource utilization performance and costs.

Diagnostic guideline. A practice guideline targeted at evaluating patients with particular symptoms for the presence of diseases that would benefit from intervention. They are also used to guide the screening of asymptomatic patient populations for early stages of disease.

Direct contract model. A health plan that contracts directly with private practice physicians rather than through an independent practice association or medical group.

Direct costs. The labor, supply, and equipment costs directly attributable to the provision of a specific service (see **indirect costs**).

Disability. In a legal context, the term means incapacity for the full enjoyment of ordinary legal rights.

Disability benefit. A payment that arises because of total or permanent disability of an insured; a provision added to a policy that provides for a waiver of premium in case of total and permanent disability.

Disability income insurance. A form of health insurance that provides periodic payments to replace income when an insured person is unable to work as a result of illness or injury.

Discharge planning. The process that assesses a patient's needs for treatment after hospitalization in order to help arrange for the necessary services and resources to effect an appropriate and timely discharge.

Discovery. The process whereby information pertinent to a legal complaint is gathered. The process includes written interrogatories (questions) and depositions, which are questions and statements given under oath. It also includes expert witness testimony, the subpoena of records, and mental and physical exams of the person.

Disease state management. A process that 1) identifies patients with chronic diseases, 2) assesses the patient's health status, 3) develops or fits the patient into a program or plan of care and 4) collects data on the effectiveness of the process. Disease management attempts to proactively intervene with treatment and education so that the patient can maintain optimal function without high cost interventions. Disease state management attempts to manage the care of chronic, at risk populations across the entire continuum of care. The common types of diagnostic categories are asthma, AIDS, cancer, chronic renal failure, congestive heart failure, diabetes, hemophilia and psychiatric conditions. Disease management may use case managers in some programs or may use physician providers to act as case managers.

Dual diagnosis. A condition of both mental disorder and substance abuse.

Dual-eligible. Describes a Medicare beneficiary who also receives the full range of Medicaid benefits offered in his or her state.

Economic evaluation. Comparative analysis of alternative courses of action in terms of both their costs and their consequences.

Economic outcome. This includes the use of health care resources (direct costs) and the inability to use the same resources for other worthwhile purposes (opportunity costs).

Effectiveness of care. The degree to which care is provided in the correct manner: that is, without error, given the current state of the art; a component of quality of care.

Efficiency of care. The degree to which care received has the desired effect with a minimum of effort, expense, or waste; a component of quality of care.

Endpoint. Refers to health events that lead to completion or termination of follow-up of an individual in a trial or cohort study.

Enrollee. An individual who has elected to contract for, or participate in, a health benefit plan for him- or herself and/or his or her dependents; a subscriber.

Evaluation and management service. A nontechnical service provided by most physicians for the purpose of diagnosing and treating diseases and counseling and evaluating patients.

Evidence. Any species of proof or probative matter, legally presented at the trial of an issue, by the act of the parties and through the medium of witnesses, records, documents, tangible objects, and the like, for the purpose of inducing beliefs in the minds of the court or jury as to the truth of their contention.

Exclusion. A specific illness or treatment that is expressly not covered by a plan or insurance contract.

Experience rating. A system used by liability insurance carriers to set premium levels based on the insured's past liability experience.

Expert consensus. Agreement in opinion of clinical and methodology experts, used, for example, to develop guidelines, indicators, and indicator thresholds.

Expert witness. A person who has special knowledge of a subject about which a court requests testimony. Special knowledge may be acquired by experience, education, observation, or study, but is not possessed by the average person. An expert witness gives expert testimony or expert evidence. This evidence often serves to educate the court and the jury in the subject under consideration.

Face validity. The extent to which the concept of the measurement appears to fit the concept of the quantity being measured.

Federally qualified HMO. An HMO that has satisfied certain federal qualifications pertaining to organizational structure, provider contracts, health service delivery information, utilization review/quality assurance, grievance procedures, financial status, and marketing information.

Fee-for-service system. A system of paying physicians for individual medical services rendered, as opposed to paying them by salary or capitation. The CPT payment system and the Medicare Fee Schedule are examples of fee for service.

Fee schedule. A list of predetermined payments for units of medical service.

Fee schedule payment area. A geographic area within which payment of a given service under the Medicare Fee Schedule will be equal. Most payment areas are analogous to payment localities under the previous CPR system (see **geographic adjustment factor**).

Fiduciary relationship. A legal relationship of confidentiality that exists whenever one person trusts or relies on another, such as a doctor-patient relationship.

Fraud. A false representation of a matter of fact (whether by words or conduct, by false or misleading allegations, or by concealment of that which should be disclosed) that deceives and is intended to deceive another so that that person shall act upon such representation to his or her legal injury.

Function goal. Directed interrelated series of processes; some functions affect patients directly (for example, most clinical processes) and others only indirectly (for example, management processes and determining practitioner competence).

Functional status. The performance of, or the capacity to perform, a variety of activities normal for people in good health. This general term is used to refer to all measures of functioning regardless of whether they refer to personal or role activities.

Gaming. Gaining advantage by using improper means to evade the letter or intent of a rule or system.

Geographic adjustment factor (GAF). The adjustment factor applied to a service's fee in the Medicare Fee Schedule to determine the correct payment in each fee schedule payment area. As defined in OBRA 89, the geographic adjustment factor for a service is created by combining three separate adjustment factors, one for each component of the Medicare Fee Schedule: physician work, practice expense, and malpractice expense are based on the same measures that underlie the GPCI.

Geographic practice cost index (GPCI). An index summarizing the prices of inputs to physicians' services in an area relative to national average prices. The GPCI, originally defined by the Urban Institute and the Center for Health Economics Research, is based on three components that reflect the opportunity cost of physician work, the cost of goods and services that make up practice expenses, and malpractice expenses. The GPCI is a single measure that combines these three components as fixed shares, whereas the GAF of the Medicare Fee Schedule allows each service to reflect different shares, creating a GAF for each service.

Global satisfaction. A composite score of three "bottom-line" survey questions relating to whether the patient would praise, return to, or recommend the hospital or provider to friends or family.

Global service. A package of clinically related services treated as a unit for purposes of billing, coding, or payment.

Global surgery policy. The payment policy in the Medicare Fee Schedule stating that the global surgical fee includes not only the procedure itself but also all related services.

Gold standard. A method of established or widely accepted accuracy for determining a diagnosis. It provides a reference point against which to measure the performance of screening or diagnostic tests.

Group-model HMO. An HMO that pays a medical group a negotiated, per capita rate, which their group distributes among its physicians, usually on a salaried arrangement (see **health maintenance organization, independent practice association, staff-model HMO**).

Group practice. Three or more physicians who deliver patient care, jointly use medical equipment and personnel, and divide income by a predetermined formula.

HCA common procedure coding system (HCPCS). A coding system based on CPT, but supplemented with additional codes; required for coding by Medicare carriers (see **coding, Current Procedural Terminology**).

Health. The state of patients when they function optimally without evidence of disease or abnormality. Also, the condition best suited to reach goals that each individual formulates on his or her own.

Health benefit plan. Any public or private organization's written plan that insures or pays for specific health care expenses on behalf of enrollees or covered persons.

Health care assessment. The process of estimating the probability of particular outcomes associated with a defined intervention and of determining patient preferences for those outcomes.

Health care organization. Health facility with organized staff that provides health-related services.

Health costs. These include the use of health care resources (direct and indirect costs) and the inability to use the same resources for other worthwhile purposes (opportunity costs).

Health decision. The actual choice(s) that can be made by health care practitioners or recipients confronted by a defined health problem. A specific decision is a choice between a primary scenario and alternate scenarios.

Health intervention. Any action taken to modify the health of an individual or collection of individuals. The intervention may pertain to disease prevention, detection, diagnosis, or management.

Health maintenance organization (HMO). A prepaid, organized health care plan. Individuals are enrolled in the plan, and services are provided through a system of affiliated providers. Comprehensive benefits are financed by prepaid premiums with limited copayments (see **group-model HMO, independent practice association, staff-model HMO**).

Health outcomes. These are outcomes that patients can experience (physically and mentally) and care about. They relate to the length and quality of life and include death, functional disability, appearance, pain, anxiety, and peace of mind. Health outcomes include the benefits of detecting disease when it is present, the false security associated with failing to detect disease when it is present, and the unfounded anxiety associated with detecting disease when it is really absent. Outcomes may be immediate (such as inconvenience, discomfort, and acute adverse effects) or delayed (subsequent changes in physiological or functional status that would not have occurred in the absence of the intervention).

Health practice. Activities of persons who actually deliver care to patients; a particular type of health intervention.

Health practitioner. Anyone who implements a health intervention (e.g. physician, nurse, public health officer).

Health problem. In the context of decision analysis and practice guidelines, a health problem is adequately specified when a particular disease, illness, or condition is described for a particular patient and provider population.

Health process intervention. Change in the conduct of health care: for example, an intervention may change the nature of the doctor-patient relationship or the manner in which health actions are documented.

Health technology intervention. Although this term is often reserved for health interventions that involve the use of particular devices, reagents, or equipment, the evaluation of performance characteristics of these technologies does not differ in any significant way from evaluation of other health interventions. Issues of sensitivity, specificity, and positive predictive value apply equally to the use of chest x-rays, stethoscopes, and questions asked in a medical history.

Heuristic technique (method). A procedure for searching out an unknown goal by incremental exploration, according to some known criterion; involves the use of feedback to improve performance.

High-risk function. A key function that exposes individual patients to a greater chance of adverse occurrences if not carried out effectively and/or appropriately; also applies to services that are inherently risky, even when effective and appropriate, because of certain patient attributes and/or newness of the service.

High-volume function. A key function that is performed frequently or affects large numbers of patients: for example, diagnostic testing.

Holistic medicine. A trend in medicine that emphasizes that the system must extend its focus beyond the physical aspects of disease or particular organs. It is concerned with the whole person and the interrelationships between the emotional, social, spiritual, and physical implications of disease and health. Also called **alternative** or **complementary medicine.**

Home health care. Health care provided in the home to aged, disabled, sick, or convalescent individuals who do not need institutional care. The most common types of home care are visiting nurse services and speech, physical, occupational, and rehabilitation therapy.

Hospice. A health care program whose purpose is to provide care, compassion, and support for patients in the final stages of illness and close to death.

Hospital alliances. Groups of hospitals allied to reduce costs by sharing services and developing group purchasing programs.

ICD-9. The International Classification of Diseases, Version 9, formulated by the World Health Organization to standardize diagnoses and the etiology of disease. The purpose was to assist with research and identify public health issues, but it has become a widely used tool to assist insurance claims organizations to identify treatment requirements.

Indemnity. Security against possible loss or damage; a predetermined reimbursement amount paid in the event of a covered loss.

Independent medical exam (IME). Used by insurers to determine an individual's diagnosis, need for continued treatment, degree and permanency of disability, or ability to return to work.

Independent practice association (IPA). An HMO that contracts with individual physicians to provide services to HMO members at a negotiated per capita or fee-for-service rate. Physicians maintain their own offices and can contract with other HMOs and see other fee-for-service patients.

Indication. Guideline that specifies when certain course(s) of action are appropriate: for example, for a specific disease or condition.

Indicator information set. Indicator-specific information composed of an indicator statement, definition of terms, indicator type, rationale, description of indicator population, indicator data collection logic, and underlying factors that may explain variations in data.

Indicator measurement tool. Used to monitor and evaluate the quality of important governance, management, and undesirable indicators.

Indicator rationale. Indicator information set component that explains why an indicator is useful in specifying and assessing the process or outcome of care measured by the indicator (see **indicator information set**).

Indicator statement. Indicator information set component that describes the function, activity, or event being assessed: for example, patients for whom percutaneous transluminal coronary angioplasty has failed (see **indicator information set**).

Indicator underlying factors. Indicator information component that delineates patient, practitioner, and organization systems factors that may explain variation in data and thereby direct quality improvement activities.

Indicator validity. The degree to which an indicator identifies events that merit further review.

Indirect costs. Costs that cannot be easily traced to particular services but that must be assigned using explicit accounting methods. Sometimes referred to as common or overhead costs (see **direct costs**).

Injury. Any wrong or damage done to another individual's person, rights, reputation, or property. Consists of damages of a permanent nature.

Inside limits. Internal control limits within the structure of overall benefits or the benefit plan; utilized to establish a maximum amount for a procedure, service, confinement, disability, calendar year, etc.

Institutional variables. Factors that make up the quality of care given to patients in an institution after adjusting for patient variables and random variation.

Internal consistency. The extent to which all items in a particular scale measure the same dimension, also called **reliability**.

Interrogatories. A series of written questions submitted to a witness or other person having information of interest to the court. The answers are transcribed and are sworn to under oath.

Iterative. Describes a process involving repetitive operational procedures. Such a process assumes that data or patient classifications are equal in their assigned values and that the endpoint should be the same given the classification. Example: patients with the same diagnosis code should have the same, or nearly the same, outcome.

Job description. A detailed description of the duties, tasks, and requirements of a job, including specific physical and mental qualifications for performance. A job description is an important tool for analyzing an insured's potential to return to his or her preinjury job and for ascertaining transferable skills.

Legal reserve. The minimum reserve a company must keep to meet future claims and obligations as calculated under a state insurance code.

Liability. Legal responsibility for failure to act, so causing harm to another person, or for actions that fail to meet standards of care, so causing another person harm.

Litigation. A contest in a court for the purpose of enforcing a right.

Long-term care. Health care provided to individuals who do not require hospital care but who need nursing, medical, and other health care services provided over time.

Long-term disability income insurance. Insurance issued to a group or an individual to provide a reasonable replacement of a portion of income lost due to a serious, prolonged illness.

Loss control. Efforts by insurers and insureds to prevent accidents and reduce losses through the maintenance and upgrading of health and safety procedures.

Loss expenses. That part of an expense (such as legal allocation fees) paid by an insurance company directly to the plaintiff in settling a particular claim.

Loss-of-time benefits. Benefits paid to help replace earned income lost through inability to work because of a disability caused by accident or illness. Weekly indemnity insurance is the type of insurance that provides such benefits.

Loss ratio. The ratio of losses to premiums for a given period.

Loss reserve. The dollar amount designated as the estimated cost of an accident at the time the first notice is received.

Malfeasance. Performance of an unlawful, wrongful act.

Malingering. The practice of feigning illness or inability to work in order to collect insurance benefits.

Malpractice. Improper care or treatment by a physician; more generally, a professional person's wrongful conduct, improper discharge of professional duties, or failure to meet standards of practice, which results in harm to another person.

Maximum benefit (overall maximum benefit). The maximum amount any one individual may receive under an insurance contract. May also refer to assigning responsibility for the payment of a claim to a second insurance carrier.

Medicaid. State public assistance programs open to persons of any age whose financial resources are insufficient to pay for health care. Provided under Title XIX of the Social Security Act of 1986.

Medical service organization (MSO). A medical group practice that provides health services for a designated population of subscribers but does not assume full responsibility for the risk or costs of the care provided.

Medicare. The hospital insurance and supplementary medical insurance systems for the aged and disabled created in 1965 by amendments to the Social Security Act.

Misfeasance. An improper performance of a lawful act, especially in a way that might cause damage or injury.

Modified job. The predisability job adapted for the insured in such a manner that it can be performed within prescribed physical or mental limitations.

Motion. A request to the court to take some action or a request to the opposing side to take some action relating to a case.

Negligence. Failure to act as an ordinary prudent person; conduct contrary to that of a reasonable person under similar circumstances.

Nonduplication clause. A clause that excludes expenses incurred to the extent that an employee or dependent receives benefits under any type of policyholder-sponsored insurance plan.

Nonfeasance. A failure to perform a task, duty, or undertaking that one has agreed to perform or that one had a legal duty to perform.

Occupational therapy (OT). A program of prescribed activities that focuses on coordination and mastery and is designed to assist the insured to regain independence, particularly in activities of daily living.

Orthotics. The field that specializes in development and use of orthopedic appliances, braces, and other devices to support weight, prevent or correct deformities, or improve the function of movable parts of the body.

Overinsurance. Insurance exceeding in amount the probable loss to which it applies. Overinsurance, which can be a serious problem, is controlled in group medical care coverage by the contractual use of nonduplication of benefits provisions (e.g., coordination of benefits).

Partial disability. A condition resulting from an illness or injury that prevents an insured from performing one or more regular job functions.

Period of disability. The period during which an employee is prevented from performing the usual duties of his or her occupation or employment or during which a dependent is prevented from performing the normal activities of a healthy person of the same age and sex. More than one cause (accident or sickness) may be present during or contribute to a single period of disability.

Permanent and total disability. A disability that will presumably last for the insured's lifetime and that prevents him or her from engaging in any occupation for which he or she is reasonably fitted.

Petition. An ex parte application to a court asking for the exercise of the court's judicial powers in relation to some matter that is not the subject for a suit or action, or a request for the authority to undertake an action that requires the sanction of the court.

Physician advisor. A physician who represents a claims administrator or utilization review organization and who provides advice on whether to certify an admission, extension of stay, or other medical service as medically necessary and appropriate.

Plaintiff. A person who brings a suit to court in the belief that one or more of that individual's rights have been violated or that a legal injury has occurred.

Pleadings. The process of litigation, whereby the plaintiff sets forth a detailed recitation of his complaint and the defendant answers; the first stage of a trial.

Preadmission authorization (or precertification). The practice of requiring those covered by a health care plan to telephone a claims department prior to hospitalization, outpatient surgery, or other significant medical procedure.

Pre-existing condition. A physical or mental condition of an insured that manifested itself prior to the issuance of the individual policy or for which treatment was received prior to such issuance.

Primary care. Basic health care provided by physicians, general practitioners, internists, obstetricians, pediatricians, and mid-level practitioners that emphasizes a patient's general health needs as opposed to specialized care. Includes basic or initial diagnosis and treatment, health supervision, management of chronic conditions, and preventative health services. Appropriate referral to consultants and community resources is an important facet of primary care.

Probationary period. The length of time a person must wait from the day of his or her entry into an eligible class or application for coverage to the date that his or her insurance becomes effective.

Professional liability. A legal concept describing the obligation of a professional person to pay a patient or client for damages caused by the professional's act of omission, commission, or negligence. Professional liability better describes the responsibility of all professionals to their clients than does the concept of malpractice, but the idea of professional liability is central to malpractice.

Profile. A longitudinal or cross-sectional aggregation of medical care data. A patient profile lists all of the services provided to a particular patient during a specified period of time. Physician, hospital, or population profiles are statistical summaries of the pattern of practice of individual physicians or hospitals or the medical experience of specific populations. Diagnostic profiles, a subcategory of physician, hospital, or population profiles, focus on a specific condition or diagnosis.

Prospective review. Utilization review conducted prior to a patient's hospital stay or course of treatment.

Provider. A licensed health care facility, physician, or other health care professional that delivers health care services.

Quality improvement (QI). See **continuous quality improvement**.

Rate. The charge per unit of payroll used to determine workers' compensation or other insurance premiums. The rate varies according to the risk classification of the policyholder.

Rating. The application of the proper classification rate and other factors that may be used to set the premium rate for a policyholder. The three principal forms are manual, experience, and retrospective rating.

Reconsideration. An initial request for additional review of a utilization review organization's determination not to certify an admission, extension of stay, or other medical service. A reconsideration request is called an **expedited appeal** by some utilization review organizations.

Rehabilitation. Restoration of a totally disabled person to a meaningful occupation. A provision in some long-term disability policies provides for a continuation of benefits or other financial assistance while a totally disabled insured is being retrained or attempting to resume productive employment.

Release. The relinquishment of a right, claim, or privilege by a person in whom it exists or to whom it accrues, to the person against whom it might be demanded or enforced.

Remedy. The means by which a right is enforced or the violation of a right is prevented, redressed, or compensated.

Reserves. An amount representing actual or potential liabilities that is kept by an insurer to cover debts to policyholders for covered services.

Res ipsa loquitur. Literally, "The thing speaks for itself." A legal doctrine that applies when the defendant was solely and exclusively in control at the time the plaintiff's injury occurred, so that the injury would not have occurred if the defendant had exercised due care. When a court applies this doctrine to a case, the defendant bears the burden of proving that he or she was not negligent.

Respondeat superior. Literally, "Let the master respond." This maxim means that an employer is liable in certain cases for the consequences of the wrongful acts of its employees while the employee is acting within the scope of his or her employment.

Review criteria. The written policies, decision rules, medical protocols, or guides used by a utilization review organization to determine certification (e.g., appropriateness evaluation protocol [AEPs] and intensity of service, severity of illness, discharge, and appropriateness [ISD-A] screens).

Right-to-access law. A law that grants a patient the right to see his or her medical records.

Right-to-die law. A law that upholds a patient's right to choose death by refusing extraordinary treatment when the patient has no hope of recovery. Also referred to as the **natural death law** or **living-will law.**

Settlement. An agreement by the parties to a transaction or controversy that resolves some or all of the issues involved in a case.

Settlement options. The provisions (stated or intended) in insurance contracts that allow an insured or beneficiary to receive benefits in other than a lump-sum payment, called **structural settlement.**

Short-term disability income insurance. Insurance that pays benefits during the time a disability exists to a covered person who remains disabled for a specified period not to exceed two years.

Staff-model HMO. An HMO that employs physicians who operate out of their own facilities or clinics but who receive a salary from the HMO.

Standards of care. A structural measure of the quality of health services. In a malpractice lawsuit, those acts performed or omitted that an ordinary, prudent person in the defendant's position would have done or not done; a measure by which the defendant's alleged wrongful conduct is compared.

Statute. The written act of a legislative body declaring, commanding, or prohibiting an action (in contrast to unwritten common law).

Statute of limitations. A statute that sets forth limitations of the right or action for certain described causes (e.g., declaring that no suit can be maintained on such cases of action unless brought within a specified period of time after the right came into existence).

Stop-loss insurance. Insurance taken by employer groups to cover the financial responsibility of health benefit payments that exceed an established threshold.

Subpoena. A process commanding a witness to appear and give testimony in court.

Subrogation. The contractual right of the plan or carrier, where state law permits, to succeed to the rights of the covered person in relation to a claim against a third party.

Targeted review. A review process that focuses on specific diagnoses, services, hospitals, or practitioners rather than on all services provided or proposed to be provided to enrollees.

Taxonomy. A system for identifying or classifying objects on the basis of their relationships; an ordering system.

Third-party administration (TPA). Administration of a group insurance plan by some person or firm other than the insurer or the policyholder.

Third-party payment. Payment of health care by an insurance company or other organization so that the patient does not directly pay for his or her services.

Tort. A private or civil wrong outside of a contractual relationship.

Tort-feasor. A wrongdoer who is legally liable for the damage caused.

Transferable skills. The skills an insured has acquired through occupational or vocational endeavors that may be applied with minimal training in another occupation.

Uniform anatomical gift act. A law of the type existing in all 50 states that allows anyone over 18 to sign a donor card willing some or all of his or her organs after death.

Utilization. Utilization is commonly examined in terms of patterns or rates of use of a single service or type of service (hospital care, prescription drugs, physician visits). Measurement of utilization of all medical services in combination is usually done in terms of dollar expenditures.

Utilization review organization. An entity that conducts utilization review and determines certification of an admission, extension of stay, or other health care service.

Vocational evaluation. A professional analysis of the insured's work potential, integrating information about physical capabilities, mental aptitudes, interests, personality motivation, transferable skills, and environmental considerations.

Waiver. The intentional or voluntary relinquishment of a known right.

Workers' compensation. The social insurance system for industrial and work injuries regulated in certain specified occupations by the federal government.

Workers' compensation law. A statute imposing liability on employers to pay benefits and furnish care to employees injured and to pay benefits to dependents of employees killed in the course of and because of their employment.

Wrongful death statute. A statute of the type existing in all states that provides that the death of a person can give rise to a cause of legal action brought by the person's beneficiaries in a civil suit against the person whose willful or negligent acts caused the death. Prior to the existence of these statutes, a suit could be brought only if the injured person survived the injury.

Wrongful life action. A civil suit usually brought against a physician or health facility on the basis of negligence that resulted in the wrongful birth or life of an infant. The parents of the unwanted child seek to obtain payment from the defendant for the medical expenses of pregnancy and delivery, for pain and suffering, and for the education and upbringing of the child. Wrongful life actions have been brought and won in several situations, including malpractice tubal ligations, vasectomies, and abortions. Failure to diagnose pregnancy in time for abortion and incorrect medical advice leading to the birth of a defective child have also led to malpractice suits for a wrongful life.

Appendix C

Acronyms

A&H	accident and health insurance
A&S	accident and sickness (insurance)
AAA	Area Agency on Aging; American Arbitration Association
AAPPO	American Association of Preferred Provider Organizations
AARP	American Association of Retired Persons
ACCC	Advanced Competency Continuity of Care
ACR	adjusted community rating
ADA	Americans with Disabilities Act
ADEA	Age Discrimination in Employment Act
ADL	activity of daily living
AEP	appropriateness evaluation protocol
AHCPR	Agency for Health Care Policy and Research
AHP	accountable health plan (or partnership)
AMA	American Medical Association
AMCRA	American Managed Care and Review Association
ANYOCC	any occupation (used in long-term disability policies)
AP	attending physician

ASO	administrative services only
BCBSA	Blue Cross Blue Shield Association
CARF	Certification Association of Rehabilitation Facilities
CBO	Congressional Budget Office
CCM	certified case manager
CHAMPUS	Civilian Health and Medical Program of the Uniformed Services
CHAP	Community Health Accreditation Program
CHPA	Community Health Purchasing Alliance
CIRS	certified insurance rehabilitation specialist
CIRSC	Certification of Insurance Rehabilitation Specialists Commission
CM	case manager
CMN	certificate of medical necessity
CMO	case management organization
CMSA	Case Management Society of America
CMSS	Council of Medical Specialty Societies
COB	coordination of benefits
COBRA	Consolidated Omnibus Reconciliation Act of 1986
CPHA	Commission on Professional and Hospital Activities
CPI	Consumer Price Index
CPR	cardio-pulmonary resusitation
CPT	Current Procedural Terminology (used in billing code designations)
CRRN	certified rehabilitation registered nurse
DME	durable medical equipment
DMERC	Durable Medical Equipment Regional Carriers
DOA	date of accident
DOL	date of loss
DRG	diagnosis-related group
EAP	Employee Assistance Program
EPO	exclusive provider organization
ERISA	Employment Retirement Income Security Act
FCE	functional capacity evaluation
FFS	fee for service

FMC	Foundation for Medical Care
GAO	Government Accounting Office
HCFA	Health Care Financing Administration
HCPC	health care procedure code
HHS	U.S. Department of Health and Human Services
HIA	health insurance alliance
HIAA	Health Insurance Association of America
HIO	health insuring organization
HIPC	health insurance purchasing cooperative
HISOCC	his occupation (used in long-term disability policies)
HME	home medical equipment
HMO	health maintenance organization
HPPC	health plan purchasing cooperative
HSQ	Health Status Questionnaire
ICD-9	International Classification of Diseases
ICMA	individual case management association
IOM	Institute of Medicine
IPA	individual practice association
ISD-A	intensity of service, severity of illness, discharge and appropriateness screens
ISSI	intensity of service, severity of illness criteria
JCAHO	Joint Commission on Accreditation of Healthcare Organizations
LOS	length of stay
LPN	licensed practical nurse
LTD	long-term disability
LVN	licensed vocational nurse
MCO	managed care organization
MSGP	multispecialty group practice
MSO	managed-service organization
NAHC	National Association for Home Care
NCQA	National Committee for Quality Assurance
NMHCC	National Managed Health Care Congress
OT	occupational therapist or occupational therapy

PCP	primary care physician
PDC	physician–developed criteria
PHO	physician–hospital organization
PIP	personal injury protection (auto policy clause)
POS	point of service
PPO	preferred provider organization
PPS	prospective payment system
PRO	peer review organization
PSRO	peer standards review organization
PT	physical therapist or physical therapy
QA	quality assurance
QI	quality improvement
RBRVS	Resource-Based Relative Value Schedule (or scale)
RFP	request for proposal
RTW	return to work
SCI	spinal cord injury
SF-36	(Medical Outcomes Study) Short Form-36
SHMO	social health maintenance organization
SIMS	surgical indications monitoring criteria
SPD	summary plan description
SSA	Social Security Administration
STD	short-term disability
TBI	traumatic brain injury
TEFRA	Tax Equity and Fiscal Responsibility Act of 1982
TPA	third-party administrator
TPN	total parenteral nutrition
UM	utilization management
UR	utilization review
URAC	Utilization Review Accreditation Commission
URO	Utilization Review Organization
VC	vital capacity
WC	workers' compensation

Index

About the Author

Michael Newell, RN, MSN, CCM, is a Consultant with the health care practice of Ernst & Young, LLP, in Iselin, New Jersey. He is a 1974 graduate of the nursing program at Philadelphia Community College, and a graduate of the master's in nursing administration program at La Salle University in Philadelphia. He attributes his call to nursing to having been the oldest of 11 children.

The bulk of Mr. Newell's nursing experience is in critical care, although he has taught clinical nursing and done hospital and external case management supervision. In 1981, he co-founded Skilled Nursing Inc., one of the first contract agencies placing highly skilled nurses in critical care units in the Philadelphia area. He has been active in nursing professional organizations, including present board-of-director positions with the Professional Rehabilitation Network, the case management society in southern New Jersey, and the Delaware Valley Health Information Management and Systems Society.

3